T0144746

# BASIC HEALTH PUBLICATIONS USER'S GUIDE

## TO NATURAL ALLERGY RELIEF

---

*Learn about the Many Ways to Reduce Your Allergies.*

JONATHAN BERKOWITZ, M.D.

JACK CHALLEM Series Editor

The information contained in this book is based upon the research and personal and professional experiences of the author. It is not intended as a substitute for consulting with your physician or other healthcare provider. Any attempt to diagnose and treat an illness should be done under the direction of a healthcare professional.

The publisher does not advocate the use of any particular healthcare protocol but believes the information in this book should be available to the public. The publisher and author are not responsible for any adverse effects or consequences resulting from the use of the suggestions, preparations, or procedures discussed in this book. Should the reader have any questions concerning the appropriateness of any procedures or preparations mentioned, the author and the publisher strongly suggest consulting a professional healthcare advisor.

Series Editor: Jack Challem
Editor: Roberta W. Waddell
Typesetter: Gary A. Rosenberg
Series Cover Designer: Mike Stromberg

Basic Health Publications User's Guides are published by Basic Health Publications, Inc.

ISBN: 978-1-59120-048-2 (Pbk.)
ISBN: 978-1-68162-862-2 (Hardcover)

# CONTENTS

# INTRODUCTION

I'm in my bed, groaning. There's a pile of soggy tissues on the floor sprouting alien life forms. Parts of my nose I didn't even know existed are running and I can't keep up with them. Two of my front teeth have been blown out from sneezing. Sound vaguely familiar? Okay, okay—I'm exaggerating, but you get the idea. I have allergies. I hate allergies.

For most people, allergies are an annoying fact of life that affect approximately 10 to 20 percent of Americans. What is responsible for such misery? While most any substance can cause an allergic reaction in a sensitized individual, the most notorious allergy offenders are animal dander, dust mites, feathers, molds, and pollen. We'll talk more about these bad boys later. It is also no secret that allergies and asthma have increased more than 25 percent in the last twenty years. Although there are a number of possible reasons for this increase, air pollution, diet, food contamination, and tobacco abuse are the leading environmental/lifestyle suspects, along with a decreased consumption of the antioxidant nutrients commonly found in fish, fruits, and vegetables, and our increased consumption of polyunsaturated fats coupled with a decreased intake of oily fish. According to one study in the journal *Thorax*, "diet has been a determinant of the worldwide increases in asthma and allergies."

As with most of life's problems, the more you know the better off you are. Allergies are no exception and the more you know about allergies, the better you'll feel. It is hoped that what you will learn from this guide will, at the very least, help you control, and perhaps even remove, allergies from your life. The first step in understanding allergies is to be clear about the word "allergy." As discussed in Chapter 1, allergies mean different things to different people and rarely are two allergies exactly alike.

Perhaps even more important is to know what triggers your symptoms. Knowing what you are allergic to (the focus of Chapter 2) is the most critical question you can answer. If you know what you're allergic to, there's a good chance you can avoid that offending agent and perhaps even rid yourself of allergy symptoms. Knowing your allergies relates directly to source control, the subject of Chapter 3. Source control means removing those items from your environment that are responsible for your symptoms. Study after study has demonstrated that source control is, without a doubt, the most effective means of allergy elimination.

What happens, however, if you can't identify your allergy triggers, or if you're allergic to pollen or ragweed, allergens that source control cannot readily eliminate? This is where diet and supplements enter the allergy picture. Chapter 4 discusses how our diet can, in part, determine how allergic we are and can even make us less allergic. Diet, coupled with supplements, herbs, and other alternative therapies (the subjects of Chapters 5 and 6), can offer relief to those with allergies for whom source control is impractical. You may first want to consult with your own physician or healthcare practitioner before beginning a new regimen.

As stated, the whole purpose of this book is to

either make your life allergy-free or, at the very minimum, reduce the amount of allergy medications you take. Yet, despite our best efforts, there will always be some people who will need powerful antiallergy pharmaceuticals to help relieve their allergic symptoms, the focus of Chapter 7. If you find you're one of these people, don't despair. Most of these medications work but may have potentially dangerous side effects. Other medications, such as Nasalcrom, are considered relatively safe and can be bought without a doctor's prescription. In the final analysis, no matter where you fit into the allergy picture, this book will lead you to ask those important questions that will help you discover what your individual allergies are and, more important, how you can control and perhaps even eliminate them.

# CHAPTER 1

# ALLERGY FACTS

The word "allergy" has different meanings for different people, but for most, it means seasonal hay fever, those fits of sneezing and runny nose that occur during predictable times of the year, such as spring or fall. For others, the word means a food or drug allergy characterized by a rash when, for example, ingesting a certain medication, or by diarrhea after eating a particular food. Some people may know exactly what triggers their allergies while, for others, the cause of their misery remains a mystery. Allergies, like people, come in all shapes and sizes, but for the vast majority of people, allergies begin with the nose.

From a functional standpoint, the nose helps us breathe, warm, moisturize, and filter air before it reaches our tender lungs. The word "allergen" is a medical term for a particle that can cause an allergic reaction. Allergens vary from person to person and can range from pollen to food additives. For the vast majority of people, however, allergens are airborne, and it is when an allergen is trapped inside the nose that our troubles begin.

Let us take a moment to examine the word "allergen." One of the important

**Allergen**
*Generic term for any inhaled or ingested particle (dander, food coloring, pollen, etc.) that can trigger an allergic reaction. The words "allergen" and "antigen" are often interchangeable.*

roles of the body's immune system is to identify "self" from "non-self." Self is what belongs to us: the cells, organs, and tissues that make up our bodies. Non-self includes the rest of the world that is not a natural part of our bodies and can include bacteria, viruses, food, and pollen; it is also referred to as allergens or antigens. The immune system's ability to differentiate self from non-self is obviously important, as antigens can represent dangerous organisms like bacteria or fungi. Most any substance can act as an antigen/allergen, but the body usually reacts hostilely only to antigens it considers harmful. This hostile reaction starts with the body's formation of antibodies, which are proteins that bind to antigens and alert the immune system that a potentially dangerous invader is present.

> **Antigen**
> *Any molecule (for example, pollen) that can interact with the immune system and trigger a response, such as an allergic reaction.*

While these antibodies are found throughout the body, for allergic people it is the antibodies residing in the nose and lungs that cause the most trouble. The nose and lungs are covered by a lining called "respiratory epithelium" that harbors many different cells and proteins, such as immunoglobulins and mast cells. Immunoglobulins are those protein antibodies that act like sentries, recognizing allergens and binding to them. Our tissues contain millions of individual antibodies that are specially manufactured to recognize a specific antigen. For instance, we have antibodies that recognize only the influenza virus. We have other antibodies that recognize only certain types of fungi. Whether or not a person develops an

> **Antibody**
> *An immune-system protein that binds to a specific allergen or antigen, and can trigger an allergic reaction. The chief antibody of the allergic response is immunoglobulin E (IgE).*

immune or allergic reaction to an antigen depends on whether or not they have antibodies specific for that antigen. Virtually every person on Earth has antibodies to the influenza virus, for example, but not to ragweed, which explains why some people are allergic to ragweed and others are not.

**Immunoglobulin**
*Protein central to immune-system response, including the allergic reaction, respon- sible for binding and identifying potential allergic triggers.*

Say, for instance, you inhale a virus. The virus has antigens on its surface that help it attach to the respiratory epithelium and allow it to be recognized by an immunoglobulin specifically designed for that virus. When the immunoglobulin binds to the virus, an antibody-antigen interaction occurs that, in turn, sounds the alarm. Once the alarm is sounded, natural killer (NK) cells rush in and decimate the invading virus.

Now, where do mast cells and allergies fit into this antibody-antigen interaction? Mast cells belong to the immune system and, when stimulated, release chemicals like histamine that cause allergy symptoms. Of all the allergy-related cells, the mast

**Histamine**
*The most important chemical mediator of the allergic response, responsible for the majority of allergy symptoms.*

cells are the ones most responsible for the allergic response, and are to blame for up to half of all allergy symptoms. Even worse, mast cells spread the message to other immune system cells, such as basophils, eosinophils, and leukocytes, to make them aware that an allergen is present. As for anti - bodies, the chief antibody of the allergic response is immunoglobulin E (IgE). It is the job of IgE to recognize and form an antibody-antigen interac- tion with allergens like pollen and dander.

As an example of how this works, let's say you have an allergy to cats. You inhale some cat dander that attaches to the respiratory epithelium of your nose where it is recognized and bound in an antigen-antibody interaction by IgE that is specific to cat dander. Once this antibody-antigen interaction occurs, the IgE lets the the local mast-cell population know what it has found. Then, once the mast cells know that there is an allergen present, they panic and send out the alarm to the basophil, eosinophil, and neutrophil cells, which, in turn, release or aid in the release of histamine, prostaglandin-2, and leukotrienes, all chemical mediators (substances) that cause sneezing, coughing, and runny nose. Bottom line? You feel miserable!

**Leukocytes**
Synonymous with white blood cells, this is a general term for any white cell that belongs to the immune system.

The concept of chemical mediators is important because the most successful allergy therapies block such inflammatory substances as histamine and leukotriene, thereby blunting or eliminating the allergic response. Many allergic reactions have two phases: an immediate phase and a delayed phase. The majority of allergic reactions occur immediately after exposure to a specific allergen, but a delayed allergic reaction can occur two to eight hours after exposure, resulting in chronic symptoms. In the first phase of the im-mediate reaction, the mast cells release histamine, but in the second, delayed phase, basophils re-lease most of the histamine. In both cases, the histamine binds to special H1 receptors that, in turn, create the signals necessary for allergy symptoms to appear.

**Leukotrienes**
Derived from arachidonic acid, these are the chief chemical mediators of the inflammatory and allergic reactions.

Unlike natural killer (NK) cells, whose primary mission is to destroy invading bacteria, the baso-phils and mast cells cause you to cough, sneeze, and drip, which is their way of helping to remove the offending allergen from your body. With food allergies, these same cells may cause diarrhea, which speeds up the removal of the irritating food. Not all anti-gens, however, cause an allergic reaction in a person. It will only be those allergens that a particu-lar individual is sensitive to that will cause an allergic reaction to occur.

**H1 Receptor**
*Binding site found on a cell membrane that specifically binds to histamine, result-ing in a cellular or allergic reaction.*

Now, just exactly what is an allergic reaction? Like allergens, allergic reactions vary from person to person, depending on how allergic they are. Some people have mild allergies characterized by a rare sneeze. Other people have severe aller-gies that cause persistent sneez-ing, coughing, headache, and runny nose. Other people have a skin reaction characterized by hives, a rash, or eczema. There is even an extreme allergic reaction called anaphylaxis that can cause potentially life-threatening airway obstruction. Mercifully, anaphylaxis is exceedingly rare and most of those with allergies are merely miserable.

**Eczema**
*General term for inflamed skin, often described as a red, itchy, raised lesion that can occasionally crust. Often caused by an allergic reaction.*

## The Allergy Bad Boys

Symptoms of a particularly miserable allergic re-sponse to the major airborne offenders (animal dander, dust mites, feathers, molds, and pollen) can include intermittent or persistent sneezing, runny nose, stuffy nose, and tearing, with itchy eyes, itchy nose, itchy throat, and itchy skin thrown in for good measure. Other common symptoms include fatigue and allergic shiners. Fatigue is per-haps the most overlooked debilitating allergy symptom, and is all too often blamed on life's daily wear and tear. Allergic shiners are dusky or dark discolorations under the eyes, caused by congestion in your veins, and giving you that "I never sleep well" look. Less common allergy symptoms include abdominal pain, coughing, headaches, joint pain, and wheezing/shortness of breath with or without asthma.

As if these symptoms weren't bad enough, there is evidence that allergies can impact the way you think and work. One study published in the *Annals of Allergies* reported that people with allergies showed "declines in verbal learning, slower decision-making, and slower psychomotor speed," which translates into decreased productivity and increased work absenteeism. Equally disturbing, another study found that allergies were responsible for fragmented sleep and chronic fatigue, which, again, negatively impact your ability to concentrate. Then, adding insult to injury, other studies have related allergies to acne, asthma, attention deficit hyperactivity disorder (ADHD), depression, irritable bowel syndrome, migraine headaches, and rheumatoid arthritis.

Allergies are divided into seasonal and perennial. Seasonal allergies usually occur during predictable times of the year and are typically caused by pollens from flowers, grasses, or trees. For instance, North American ragweed tends to release pollen from mid-August to mid-October, and ragweed-sensitive people feel particularly rotten during this period. A similar scenario exists for trees that release pollen from March to May, and for grasses that pollinate from June to mid-July.

Instead of feeling rotten only at certain times of the year, people with perennial allergies get to feel miserable year round. Perennial allergies usually develop during adulthood, and women are more frequently affected than men. The condition is often associated with nasal polyps, the biggest offenders being animal dander, cockroach droppings, and dust mites. Molds are another major player in the allergy wars and they can cause seasonal or perennial allergies. Occasionally, some individuals have increasing allergic aggravations after inhaling cigarette smoke or after a sudden temperature change.

While the above lists the most common allergic triggers, anything can act as an allergen in a sensitized individual. For instance, while many allergic people have allergies to pollen or animal dander, most people with allergies exhibit multiple allergic triggers to a diverse array of products, from laundry detergent to poison ivy or air pollution. As I said, in a sensitive individual, anything can trigger an allergic response.

As long as we're talking bad boys, let's define the word "dust." You hear many people blaming their allergies on "dust." Let me tell you that no one is allergic to "dust," rather they are allergic to something in that dust, such as dander, dust mites, or pollen. In fact, many parents often blame a blanket, a piece of clothing, or a toy for a child's allergies when it is really the dust contained in the textiles that is causing the symptoms.

## Allergies—Why Me?

Allergies are an equal opportunity condition, sharing their misery with all ages, races, and sexes. While anyone can have allergies, and allergies can develop anytime between infancy and old age, we know they tend to be worse during childhood and become less severe with advancing age. Environment clearly plays a role, not only for your typical pollen-induced runny nose, but also, according to one study, by your living in an urbanized area, which was "a significant predictor of asthma and rhinitis." You can also blame your parents because allergies tend to run in families. On the whole, though, aller

**Rhinitis**
*Inflammation of the nose's internal lining. This is one of the most common allergy symptoms.*

gies represent a complex interplay between genes and environment, a finding that is echoed by studies done on twins. Clearly, some people inherit their allergies, but there are many people with allergies who belong to families in which no allergic disease can be identified.

Nevertheless, the single greatest risk factor for allergies is atopy, an exaggerated allergic reaction to the environment that often runs in families. This condition affects approximately 30 percent of the population and can cause allergic rhinitis, asthma, eczema (for example, eczematous dermatitis), food allergies, hay fever, or hives (for example, urticaria). Atopic people usually have allergies or have family members with asthma and/or allergies. The airways of allergic people with atopy tend to respond more intensely to allergens (cat dander, for example) than the airways of allergic people without atopy.

The allergic reactions found in atopic individuals can range from seasonal hayfever to eczema and asthma. People with atopy also often have elevated immunoglobulin E (IgE) in their blood, a chief mediator (substance) of the allergic reaction.

**Urticaria**
*Commonly called hives or wheals (welts), this is usually a raised, swollen, and itching skin lesion that can be caused by drugs, food, or other allergic triggers.*

And, as I said above, to make matters worse, atopic people have an exaggerated response to allergens that, in most people, the immune system would regard as harmless. In fact, unlike most allergic people, atopic people need only a very small amount of an allergen to trigger their allergic response.

## Food and Drug Allergies

Besides those people with allergies caused by animal dander, dust mites, or pollen, there are some people who are allergic to foods or drugs. In a susceptible individual, almost any food can cause an allergic reaction, but the classic offenders are dairy products, eggs, and peanuts. Drug allergies can be especially dangerous because medications are taken internally for maximal effect, and in rare instances, the allergic reaction to them can be lifethreatening. This does not mean that, if you have allergies, you shouldn't take any medications. If you've been taking a particular medication without any harmful side effects for the last twenty years, now is not the time to stop. You should, however, be aware that drug allergies do exist and they can cause allergic symptoms.

While experts agree that most allergens are airborne, food allergies do play a role in allergic disease and can cause a variety of allergy-related symptoms, such as itching and eczema. In fact, it is estimated that 1 to 2 percent of adults and 8 percent of children have food allergies, and many experts suspect that eczema and other forms of skin reactions in children are frequently triggered by food allergies. Nor is it uncommon to also see food allergies in people who have seasonal or perennial allergies. Food allergies are complicated and can be caused by the food itself or by something in the food, such as a coloring or preserving agent. Since artificial coloring is commonly used, it is important to read food and drug labels to see if any is present. Other common allergy triggers are sulfiting agents used as preservatives that are frequently found in food and medicine. Common sulfiting agents include potassium bisulfite, potassium metabisulfite, sodium bisulfite, sodium sulfite, and sulfur dioxide. Beware—sulfites can hide anywhere, from the salad bar to your favorite wine.

Testing for food allergies can range from the

traditional "scratch and prick" technique to the more complicated food elimination diet. Elimination diets are used once a particular food is suspected of producing allergic symptoms. The food is subsequently completely removed from the diet and the person is observed to see if their symptoms improve. Although elimination diets can help identify an offending allergen, due to the complexities of food allergies, they are rarely sufficient to definitively diagnose a food allergy.

There is evidence that a "hypoallergenic diet" may help prevent atopic disease in infants, with one study reporting that "90 percent of infants with allergic rhinitis and/or bronchial asthma im-

**Allergic Rhinitis**
*Inflammation of the lining of the nose, a common allergy-related symptom associated with hay fever.*

proved on a hypoallergenic diet." Hypoallergenic diets rely on prolonged breastfeeding, with the mother avoiding cow's milk, eggs, and fish for three months. This regimen has been shown to reduce the incidence and severity of atopic disease in children up to the age of five.

There is also evidence that avoiding sugars and food additives can help reduce the incidence and severity of atopic illnesses, including food allergies. The reasons why breastfeeding can protect against atopic disease remain a mystery, but researchers think that there are substances in breast milk that inhibit IgE, so breastfeeding may help the infant's mucosal defenses to mature. While eliminating a food allergy may not entirely cure your allergy problem, it can help you feel better and experience a general improvement in health.

## Medical Conditions That Mimic Allergy

Perhaps the most common medical condition that can mimic allergies is asthma. In fact, increased constriction in the airway is a common finding in people with allergies, with or without asthma. Nevertheless, asthma and allergies often go hand in hand and it is no secret that people with asthma frequently have allergies and vice versa.

Nose and throat anatomy are occasionally to blame for allergylike symptoms, as is the common cold. Some people experience nasal irritation when they inhale chemicals or perfumes. Pregnancy can also be associated with a chronic stuffy nose that may masquerade as an allergy. Vasomotor rhinitis is a condition caused by an overactive nose and is frequently misdiagnosed as an allergy. Finally, certain medications like beta-blockers, estrogens, and nose drops can cause allergylike symptoms.

**Rhinorrhea**
*Thin mucous discharge from the nose. This is one of the most common symptoms of allergic rhinitis.*

## Diagnosing Allergies

Most practitioners know if you have allergies by taking a simple history and giving you a physical examination. The most important thing you need to know is what is causing your allergies. Most practitioners, conventional or integrative (as I am—integrative medicine is a relatively new and growing field that combines conventional treatment with complementary/alternative approaches), can prescribe a drug or a supplement. It's easy to treat a symptom, but much more difficult to prevent it. This is why you should be tested for specific allergens—so you know what to avoid. Avoiding an allergen is always the best medicine.

With respect to allergy testing, the tried and true "scratch and prick" skin test is a good test. Basically, the practitioner will introduce a small amount of allergen just below your skin to see if a reaction develops. While there exists super-fancy enzyme-linked immunosorbent assay (ELISA) tests, most people need no more than the simple scratch and prick.

An important point to remember is that many of those with allergies are sensitive to multiple allergens. While scratch and prick testing can identify multiple allergic triggers, it is rarely possible to discover every allergen sensitivity in a particular person. So, even though allergy testing may not be able to identify everything you're allergic to, it will find the most common triggers, and with the help of this book, you can use this knowledge to improve your life.

Remember, when you go in for testing, you should ask if there are any other medical conditions that may be responsible for your symptoms. As mentioned earlier, conditions like asthma, vasomotor rhinitis, and even pregnancy can cause allergylike symptoms. At that time, you should also ask if there are any medications or foods that may be causing your symptoms.

# CHAPTER 2

# WHAT ARE YOU ALLERGIC TO?

**K**nowledge is power, and this is especially true for allergies. Learning about allergies and knowing what you are allergic to is the first step in leading an allergy-free life. Most people with allergies can identify several things they know will trigger a reaction. Finding these triggers and eliminating them from your environment is a critical step in making you allergy-free. I hope that, after reading this chapter, some of you will quickly find that magic trigger and rid yourself of allergies. Most people, however, myself included, will have to do some detective work. There will be some trial and error, but if you are patient and methodical, you will discover what makes your allergies tick and be able to conquer them.

I'm sure most of you can name five to ten things that set off your nose or stomach. The most important task for an allergy detective is to ask these five basic questions each time you have an attack:

**1.** Where am I?

**2.** What am I doing?

**3.** What is around me?

**4.** Do I know what set off this attack or not?

**5.** How severe is this attack?

After you answer these questions, take out your "Allergy Diary"—an allergy journal I would like you to use to record the answers to these questions, along with the date and time of the attack. Everyone has their own style of keeping an allergy diary, but the following headings will help you immensely in determining what triggers your symptoms:

- Date/Time: What date and time did the attack start?

- Location/Activity: Where were you and what were you doing at the start of the attack?

- Trigger: What triggered the attack? If you only suspect a trigger, put a "?" next to it.

- Severity: How severe were your symptoms? Use a mild-moderate-severe scale.

- Treatment/Interventions: How did you get rid of your symptoms? Did you remove the offending agent from the environment, or did you remove yourself from the offending environment?

- Duration of Attack: How long did the attack last from the time you first noticed symptoms to the time you believed the attack was over?

Keeping an allergy diary may seem like a nuisance, but it will play a crucial role in helping you determine what triggers your allergies. When you record this information, I hope you will see patterns begin to develop. You may find that your allergies tend to be worse in a certain room, when performing a particular activity, or during a certain time of the year. I also want you to share your diary with a trusted friend or two and a knowledgeable professional. You never know what a fresh eye may uncover.

## Interrogation Time

Okay, it's time to ask some hard questions to dis - cover what triggers your allergies. First though, take a moment and write down five to ten things that you know trigger your allergies. For instance, one day my wife bought some wonderful flowers! Only problem was that those flowers immediately triggered a sneezing attack in me so, needless to say, those flowers will never see the inside of my home again. I want you to take this same unyielding approach to your allergy triggers. If you know something triggers an attack, you either trash it or avoid it!

This technique is called "source control," and is the single most effective way to treat allergies. As you answer the following questions, you'll find that some allergy triggers are easy to identify and remove, while others may take some investigation and involve hard decisions. The most important thing you can do right now is eliminate those triggers that you are certain precipitate an attack, and stay true to your allergy diary.

What follows is a list of questions that offers an excellent way to start you thinking about your allergies and what sets them off.

## Where Do You Live? What Do You Do?

*Do you live in the city, country, or suburbs?* Cockroaches are notorious allergy triggers and city folk shouldn't underestimate the tenacity of a cockroach or overestimate the cleanliness of their building. City dwellers also often have to contend with outdoor air pollution. For country folk, agriculture and pollen are frequent troublemakers. People who live in the suburbs often have to contend with all three: agriculture, air pollution, and pollen, if not cockroaches. No matter where you live, pay attention to the sources of indoor and outdoor air pollution.

*Do you live in an apartment or condominium?* Think about cockroaches and also about your neighbor's dog that spreads dander throughout the building. Keeping your home meticulously clean and free of dust goes a long way in reducing your allergy symptoms.

***Do you have a garden?*** Does your nose run every time your petunias sprout? You or your neighbor may have a pretty garden acting as a pollen factory. If your allergies are worse in your garden, it should be pretty obvious what's causing the problem. Moist soil and blooming flowers have this nasty habit of spewing forth fungi and pollen that are just looking for a nice nose to land in. Rather than paving your yard with asphalt, though, you might consider a Japanese rock garden, or think about growing non-pollinating, allergy-friendly plants. If you can't live without flowers, keep the windows facing your garden closed, especially during pollen season.

***What type of work do you do?*** Occupational allergies are common and the list of triggers is almost endless. The typical sad story is of the person whose allergies are worse at work but get a little bit better at home and a lot better on vacation, only to return when at work. Work-related allergies are a politically sensitive subject that can potentially put you at odds with your employer. If you do suspect your workplace is causing your symptoms, you need to make a list of the materials you work with and go over it with a healthcare professional. The best-case scenario is that you'll find what's triggering your allergies and have it removed without a hassle. The worst case scenario involves attorneys and/or changing jobs, even careers.

***What are your hobbies?*** You never know, some people's hobbies involve hidden allergy triggers. Ask yourself if your allergies feel better or worse while you are enjoying your hobby.

## What Time of Day, Week, or Year Are Your Allergies Worse?

*Are your allergies worse during a certain time of year?* If your symptoms are worse during the spring or fall, you have seasonal allergies. These boil down to a pollen problem and the recommendations found in Chapter 3 are particularly helpful for seasonal and perennial allergies.

*Are your allergies worse during the morning or night?* Bedtime symptoms may mean a dust-mite allergy. If you notice your allergies acting up during a certain time of day, think about where you are and what you're doing at that time.

*Do your allergies improve over the weekend?* If your allergies get better over the weekend, especially when away from work, you may have occupational allergies. Occupational allergies can be caused by anything: your coworker's cologne or the materials you work with. For example, some people are sensitive to wood dust. If you are, and you're in construction, that can be a big problem.

*Do your allergies get better or go away when you're on vacation?* An allergy-free vacation means that something in your home, workplace, or local environment is triggering your allergies. Your mission: to identify this something and do your best to remove it from your environment.

## Where Are Your Allergies Worse?

*Are your allergies worse at home?* Some people have allergies only at home. If this applies to you, start a room-by-room search to see where your allergies are worse. Performing a complete home search for allergy triggers is very important and is the focus of Chapter 3 where we will learn that home sweet home is jam-packed with a horrific array of allergy precipitators.

**Are your allergies worse in the bedroom?** Dust mites are known to cause allergies in sensitized individuals and are found in the best bedrooms of America. See Chapter 3 for tips on dust-mite control.

**Are your allergies worse in the kitchen?** The kitchen is home to cooking, and its food smells can drive some people's allergies nuts!

**Are your allergies worse in the bathroom?** The bathroom is another hot spot for allergy intrigue, with its steady supply of scented soaps, perfumes, cleaning agents, and mold, all of which can trigger an allergy attack.

**Are your allergies worse in the garage?** Besides auto fumes, there are pesticides, chemicals, and cleaning agents found in many garages that can all cause trouble. Properly dispose of those chemicals and cleaners you don't use, and tightly cap the others.

**Are your allergies worse in the living room?** Just when you thought there might be an allergy-safe room in the house, I have to disappoint you by saying that the living room is another major allergy troublemaker. Living rooms are usually packed with carpeting, draperies, and fluffy furniture, which all act as pollen and allergen traps that can release their allergy-provoking nectar into the air.

**Are your allergies worse in your child's room?** Children bring all sorts of stuff home, including their aversion to tidiness. Besides being a favorite hangout for authorized and unauthorized pets, your child's room probably has the dustball that ate Chicago hiding under the bed. Keep your child's room just as clean as the rest of your home.

**Are your allergies worse in the laundry room?** The personal bane of my existence, the laundry room is filled with scented fabric softeners and laundry detergents. Give your nose a trial of scent-free laundry products and see if your allergies get better.

*Do you have any indoor plants?* Besides releasing pollen, damp soil is a breeding ground for mold, a known allergy irritant.

*Are your allergies worse or better when you're at someone else's house?* If your allergies are worse at a friend's house, try to think about what they have that you don't. Do they have a pet? Do they smoke? Is it your neighbor's perfume? If your allergies are better at a friend's house, try to think what you have that your friend doesn't.

*Are your allergies worse in the car?* Do you leave your car's vent open when in traffic, thereby allowing exhaust fumes into your car? Keep your windows closed, and make sure your car's air conditioning is well maintained because mold can contaminate dirty air-conditioning systems. Always remember to close your car's windows and use its air conditioning during allergy season or on hot humid days, especially when there are air-quality alerts.

## Do People Trigger Your Allergies?

*Are your allergies worse when you're around a certain person—a boss, a friend, or a family member?* Obviously that's no excuse to avoid your boss, but consider that it could be her perfume or his cologne that's setting off your allergies. Suspect common things, such as grooming products. Although they are often overlooked sources of allergy trouble, personal-grooming products are notorious for causing allergy-related rashes.

*Are your allergies worse around your wife, hus-*

**band, or significant other?** You probably would not have married that person if their presence had triggered an allergic reaction at the outset, so whatever is giving you trouble now is probably something like a new cologne or perfume, hair product, makeup, or soap.

**Are your allergies worse around your children?** Before you know it, your child grows up and starts using adult grooming products. If, all of a sudden, your allergies act up around her or him, it's time to ask some questions.

**Are your allergies worse around a pet?** If they are, you have lots of company because, for most allergic people, pets and allergies don't mix. We'll talk more about pets in Chapter 3, but for now think hard about your pet and its impact on your health.

## What Are You Eating or Taking?

**Are your symptoms worse after you eat?** Food allergies are surprisingly common. Do you have allergic symptoms after breakfast, lunch, or dinner? If so, keep a food diary along with your allergy diary to see if there is an association between what you eat and how you feel.

**What medications are you taking?** Carefully review your prescription and over-the-counter medications with your doctor. Many medicines contain preservatives or dyes that are notorious allergy-aggravators. Also, carefully examine the ingredients of natural remedies, such as vitamins, minerals, and herbs, as they can occasionally surprise you.

## What Are Your Daily Activities?

**Are your symptoms worse in the shower?** Scented soaps and shampoos can cause allergy trouble. The shower is also a favorite breeding ground for mold, so keep your shower and bathroom mildew-free. Bathrooms, and the products they contain, are notorious for causing both inhalation-related allergies and allergic skin rashes.

*Are your allergies worse in bed?* Could be those pesky dust mites again that we will learn more about in Chapter 3.

*Does vacuuming make your allergies worse?* Among other things, carpets trap cat dander, pollen, and that infamous "dust." This is why carpets, especially wall-to-wall carpeting, are taboo and do not belong in your home.

*Does making the bed trigger your allergies?* If making the bed drives your nose wild, this almost certainly means you're sensitive to dust mites and in dire need of the help you can find in Chapter 3.

*Does dusting or cleaning furniture trigger an attack?* Glass and furniture cleaners are packed with chemicals that can provoke an attack or cause a rash. If your allergies act up during household cleaning, try switching cleaners, or have someone clean for you. If you must clean, wear rubber or latex gloves and a facemask.

## How Your Healthcare Professional Can Help Find Your Allergy Triggers

I hope that by answering these questions, you now have a better idea about what triggers your allergies. Although this is a self-help book and its purpose is to help you help yourself, at the outset I strongly urge you to speak to your healthcare professional who can be especially helpful in analyzing your allergy journal and testing you for conditions that may be causing your symptoms. At the very minimum, I suggest you get tested for food, seasonal, and pet or dust-mite allergies.

And be aware that testing positive for a specific allergen does not mean this particular allergen is causing all your symptoms because most people with allergies are sensitive to multiple allergens.

Testing positive *does* mean you are sensitive to that specific allergen and you should do what you can to avoid it. The best way to treat allergies is to try and meticulously avoid known triggers, although this may not be possible for those who have multiple allergies, or triggers like pollen. Allergy testing is only a small part of the allergy puzzle, with diet and creating an allergy-free environment completing the picture.

# CHAPTER 3

# INTERIOR DESIGN FOR ALLERGY RELIEF

According to the National Jewish Center for Immunology and Respiratory Medicine, "The most predictable health benefit will be achieved by eliminating the source of the allergen from the home—be it a pet or a heavily mite-infested sofa—or by environmental control measures designed to decrease the exposure of mite allergen."

## Home Sweet Home!

Sorry, but home may not be sweet if you have allergies. Home harbors all sorts of dust and bugs that can make you miserable. Topping the list of offenders are cats, dogs, and dust mites, but let's not forget detergents, gardens, and smoke. While it is common knowledge that outdoor air pollution contributes to allergies, it is a less well-known fact that indoor air pollution also plays a very important role. This is particularly true in the airtight energy-efficient homes that excel at trapping polluted indoor air. Add to this wall-to-wall carpeting, coupled with a healthy dust-mite population, and it's not surprising that indoor air is frequently filled with more allergens than outdoor air.

## Source Control, Ventilation, and Filtration

When it comes to allergies, the best defense is to remove the offending agent. This is known as source control. For some irritants, such as pollen, source control may be impractical or impossible, so here is where ventilating, filtering, and damp-mopping enter the picture. Unless you have the misfortune to live next to a petrochemical plant, the air outside your home is probably cleaner than the air inside your house. You can change this by opening your home's windows every day, and turning on the bathroom and kitchen exhaust fans to exchange the dirty inside air for the cleaner air outside. After you have ventilated your home for ten to thirty minutes, you can shut your windows, turn on your air conditioner or filter, and breathe a breath of fresh air.

Don't, however, ventilate your home when there are air-quality alerts; rather, let your air conditioner do the dirty work, particularly if the weather is hot and muggy. During warm summer months, use your air conditioner liberally. Air conditioners are excellent for people with allergies, because they circulate indoor air and keep humidity levels low, in the process creating a hostile environment for mold growth. If you're sensitive to pollen or mold, keep your windows closed during the high pollen/mold-count days.

If you have seasonal allergies, or are sensitive to outdoor air pollution, there may be irritants in the good outdoor air that will not make your allergies happy. This is where air cleaners/purifiers enter the picture. Particle filters range from that funny-looking boxed filter on your furnace to the high-tech, High Energy Particulate Air (HEPA) filters that remove 99.97 percent of airborne particles. The newest machines available are the "electronic precipitators," or electronic air cleaners. Using less electricity and operating noiselessly, these electronic air cleaners employ a charged filter to collect particles. Many manufacturers add ionizers that place a charge on airborne particles before they enter the system, which makes them sticky and improves their collection efficiency. Electronic air cleaners can be used alone or in combination with a HEPA filter. Avoid units that produce ozone, as this gas can irritate your lungs.

The two most important qualities of air filters are efficiency and ventilation. Efficiency relates to the percentage of airborne contaminants removed by the filter, and the HEPA filter is the standard. Ventilating power means the unit can filter a volume of air within a certain period of time, usually expressed as cubic feet per minute (cfm). Ventilating power is important because you want to clean all the air in a room within a reasonable period of time. Ideally, you want a highly efficient unit that has the ventilating power needed to filter the air in your room several times an hour.

Deciding to purchase a high-efficiency HEPA filter with a rapidly ventilating unit is easy. The hard part is deciding between the purchase of a portable/modular air cleaner and refitting your entire heating, ventilation, and air-conditioning system (HVAC) with an induct filtration unit. If you have central air conditioning or forced air heat, its ductwork essentially monopolizes the air you breathe. Even if you don't have central air conditioning or forced air heat, your home prob-ably has some type of ventilation system. While the best way to rid the air of allergens remains source control and ventilation, these measures are sometimes impractical or impossible, such as with seasonal allergies, and this is when you should consider HVAC. If you think these induct air-purifying systems sound right for you, call your local HVAC specialist.

## Portable Air Cleaners

What happens if you rarely use your furnace or air conditioner? What happens if you passed out when you learned how much an induct system costs? What do you do if you live in ductless home? The nice part about portable air cleaners is that you turn them on and, with the exception of an occasional filter change, basically ignore them. The bedroom is a logical place to start because we spend one-third of our lives in bed and because, as we will learn, the bedroom is one of the most hostile environments for allergies.

Air cleaners, however, are only a small part of the allergy solution. For an air cleaner to work, allergens must be airborne so they can enter the cleaning unit and be filtered. The problem is, most allergens, dander for example, are rarely airborne and spend most of their life trapped in your bed, carpet, or furniture. The only hope an irritant can ever have of finding its way into your nose is by being subjected to the mechanical disruption necessary for it to become airborne, such as when you make the bed, vacuum, or walk. Air purifiers are limited in their ability to reduce allergen loads because most allergens hide in textile products and are not airborne. This is why excluding carpeting, draperies, and other allergen traps from the homes of allergic people is recommended.

## Carpeting, Draperies, Furniture, and Household Cleaning

Ideally, if you have allergies, your home should be carpet-free. If you have linoleum, stone, tile, or wood floors, dump your vacuum cleaner and damp-mop them regularly. If a carpet is essential for you, I suggest that you put down area rugs instead and make sure they are cleaned monthly. If that is not acceptable, and you either will not or cannot remove your wall-to-wall carpeting, I recommend keeping it meticulously clean by vacuuming it at least once a week and turning yourself into a source-control fanatic. For textile window treatments, apply the same cleaning tips as for carpets, and treat your draperies with an anti-mildew/mite agent.

Vacuuming a carpet is perhaps one of the most dangerous activities you can perform. Every time you vacuum, you disperse into the air millions of bits of particulate pollution that is just looking for a warm, moist home like your nose. Complicating the problem is that standard vacuum-cleaner bags and "water-based" vacuum cleaners only do a mediocre job at trapping particles. Fortunately, there are high-efficiency vacuum cleaners with HEPA filters.

Ideally, people with allergies should not vacuum. If, however, you have to vacuum, make sure you ventilate your home, as you should also do when changing bed linens, or cleaning furniture, draperies, or flooring.

Along with carpets, stuffed furniture is another allergy trouble spot and can trap allergens. Although leather, vinyl, and wood furniture are more allergy friendly, you may not choose to entirely rid your home of textiles unless you have a special love for leather or vinyl.

## Humidity

Dust mites, fungus spores, and mold are a major problem for people with allergies. Keeping your home's humidity level between 30 and 50 percent can significantly reduce the mold and dust-mite populations. Air conditioners work wonders in the summer by keeping humidity levels low, and in the winter, humidity can be controlled with a dehumidifier. The bathroom is a humidity trouble spot, and it is very important to thoroughly ventilate your bathroom daily, especially after taking a shower or bath. Remember to regularly empty water trays for the air conditioner, dehumidifier, and refrigerator to keep your home's humidity levels low.

You don't need to be intimated by humidity be -

cause there are inexpensive humidity gauges that help you keep your home's humidity between 30 and 50 percent. Humidity is easy to control. If you live in the desert, you probably need a humidifier. If you live in the soggy Pacific Northwest, a dehumidifier is in your future. For everyone else, air conditioning coupled with removing obvious sources of humidity will go a long way toward keeping your home mold-free. Remember to clean your humidifier/dehumidifier regularly because a dirty unit can not only make your mold problem much worse, but can also promote contamination by potentially dangerous bacteria.

## The Bedroom

We think of the bedroom as a refuge, a place to repose, safe, in a deep slumber, but, in fact, the bedroom is often the most dangerous room in the house, primarily because it contains that dreaded piece of furniture—the bed. Besides being awakened by your snoring spouse, while you sleep you and your loved one are actually shedding skin. While you may be thinking this is not the most savory thing to contemplate, the dust mite is thinking just the opposite. Shed skin is dust-mite food, and dust mites are a fact of life that have nothing to do with how clean you keep your home. Somehow, I suspect the idea of sleeping on concrete isn't appealing to you, so I suggest you cover your box spring, comforters, mattress, and pillows in special fabrics called encasements that are designed to minimize the amount of dust-mite allergens. If you can't find encasements locally, they are available at suppliers of allergy-related products, such as The Allergy Buyers Club, Allergy Supply Company, and Allergy One, listed at the end of this book.

Since dust mites gravitate to your sheets and blankets as well as to your mattress, you can make a serious dent in their food supply by washing your blankets, comforters, mattress pads, pillow covers, and sheets every ten to fourteen days in hot (130°F) water.

Another bedroom taboo for allergic people are feathers found in pillows and those nice, soft down comforters. If your allergies are worse in the bedroom, you may want to trade in your feathered pillows and comforters for synthetic hypo-allergenic-filled items.

## The Bathroom, Kitchen, and Laundry Room

If you are sensitive to smells or have eczema, the bathroom can be scary with its variety of scented grooming products that can cause rashes and allergy symptoms in sensitive individuals. Exile your toiletry collection to the garage or outside storage shed over a weekend, when you can avoid the public, and see how your allergies behave. Ideally, one week without toiletries will give your nose and skin time to recover. After seven days, gradually reintroduce these items back into your life and see how your allergies react.

The kitchen is another allergy trouble spot with its smoke and fumes. In addition to using an exhaust fan, keep your kitchen windows open and doors closed when cooking. The kitchen is also a favorite hangout for the crumb-loving cockroach. You can avoid the ubiquitous roach by keeping your kitchen spotless and roach-proofing your home. This means no open food products in your cabinets or refrigerator for the roach to dine on. When I lived in New York City, I kept the cockroach population at bay by storing all my food in tightly sealed plastic or glass containers.

The laundry room is home to fabric softeners, scented laundry detergent, and gobs and gobs of dust, all potential red-flag items for anyone with allergies. Like the rest of your home, keep the laundry room meticulously clean and dust-free. Always shut the laundry-room door when washing or drying clothes, and if there is a door between the laundry room and the garage, keep both that door and the garage door open to allow the dust and fumes to escape. Until you figure out exactly what does and does not trigger your allergies, I recommend you stick with unscented detergents and fabric softeners.

## Outdoor Clothing

Ideally, in order to reduce the amount of dander and other allergens finding their way into your home, any item of clothing that is worn outdoors should not be brought into the house. You're probably saying, "But I don't have a pet!" Doesn't matter. Just ask the Swedes who conducted studies on school dust and found that it contained high levels of dog and cat allergens (obviously a surprise to the superintendent who thought he was running a school, not a kennel). Apparently, the dander was being brought into the school on the children's clothing and shoes. Moral of the story: if you think your home is safe from dog and cat dander, think again. Cat/dog dander is everywhere, floating through the air and landing, guess where? On your clothes!

Every time you come home, you track in pollen and dander on your clothes that your nose would be better off without. So, if possible, keep items like shoes or coats either outdoors or in the garage. If this is impractical, then designate one closet near an entrance to the house as the repository of all outdoor clothing, and whatever you do, don't allow any outdoor garment or shoes to go beyond this closet and deeper into the house.

## Your Child's Room

I don't need to tell you that neatness and children

often don't mix, but if you or your child have allergies, it's in everybody's best interest to make sure your child's room stays as clean as the rest of the house. Even if your children don't have allergies, I would still encase and regularly wash their bedding since the dust mites also feed on your children's skin. Every now and then, check under your child's bed to see how big the dust-ball collection is getting, and do a quick room search for unauthorized pets. As your child gets older, don't be surprised if an interest in romance develops, an interest often heralded by the sudden appearance of allergy-provoking scented products.

## Plants and Gardens

When gardening, place a mask over your face so you don't inhale soil and plant allergens. Overgrown plants and shrubs are potential allergy offenders and should be kept neat. Needless to say, if you're allergic to grass, it pays to have a neighborhood youth mow your lawn. Other sources of allergy trouble are houseplants that may aggravate your allergies by releasing pollen or by serving as a breeding ground for molds.

## Pets

You probably love your pet as much as you love your family, but whether you're a cat or dog lover, the truth is that pets are a leading contributor to allergic illness. Both cats and dogs can cause allergy trouble, but of the two, it's the cat that poses the most danger because feline dander is smaller and therefore more likely to remain airborne. Allergy skin testing can help determine if your pet is part of the problem, especially if you have a strong reaction, but be aware that skin testing can be inaccurate and does not always test for pet-related products.

This is where keeping an allergy diary becomes

critically important. If you find that your allergies improve when the dog is away, then perhaps he or she is the problem and a trial separation is needed. Leave your pet with a trusted friend or a pet-care professional for one month and completely remove all pet products from your home. You'll also need to eliminate residual dander by thoroughly cleaning your home and washing all clothes, linens, and carpeting. This trial separation may be painful, and if, after four weeks, your symptoms don't improve, chances are your pet isn't to blame. On the other hand, if your allergies miraculously disappear with your pet, then you have a hard decision to make.

If you can't give up your pet, you should seriously consider keeping her or him forever outdoors, along with any pet-related products. If you cannot do this, then at least restrict your pet to as few rooms as possible. Make one room a pet room, making sure the space is adequately ventilated, has an air cleaner/purifier, and is damp-mopped weekly, at least. Also, make sure your home has several HEPA filter devices that can significantly reduce the animal dander load. Make sure, too, that whatever your pet sleeps on is laundered weekly and, whatever you do, never let your pet sleep with you. In fact, keep your pet out of the bedroom altogether. Wash your pet twice weekly, since a clean pet leaves behind less dander. There are actually pet-care products, such as PetWize (cat and dog allergen control you apply to your pet's fur to reduce dander), that help. One British study found that washing your pet twice a week reduced airborne dog allergens by 84 percent.

## What Are You Going to Do Today?

The whole purpose of this chapter is to create an allergy-safe environment through source control. I cannot guarantee that by following this advice you will rid yourself of allergies. I do, however, suspect that the majority of those who follow this advice will experience a significant improvement in their symptoms and life. What you need to do now is formulate an action plan to create an allergy-safe environment.

Search your entire home, room by room, and make a list of all potential allergens, such as chemicals, cleaning agents, and personal-care products. Immediately discard outdated items or ones you don't use. Once you have a list, set a date on which, in one fell swoop, you rid your home of as many allergens as possible. On that same day, have your entire home cleaned from top to bottom, preferably by a professional cleaning company. Pay special attention to textile products because they are notorious allergen reservoirs. Remember, even if your dog is on vacation, his dander is not; it's hiding in your carpet and furniture. Have all area rugs, comforters, draperies, and window treatments professionally laundered. If you have a roach problem, carefully examine your kitchen and identify trouble spots. You may need to hire an exterminator.

Inform your family of your plans. Allergies are not just your problem, they are everyone's problem, and you'll need your family's support and cooperation, especially after telling your daughter her hairspray is banished for a week. And be aware that, while your family cares about your health, temptation is everywhere, so don't be surprised if your son smells of cologne on date night. Chances are, though, that after a couple of days, you will feel better. Once your allergies have calmed down, then you can gradually reintroduce cleaning and personal-care products into your home, making sure to carefully record your symptoms. Don't be surprised if you find that one or two very common household items are provoking an allergic reaction. If that is the case, these products should be ousted as soon as possible.

# CHAPTER 4

# ALLERGIES AND DIET—YOU ARE WHAT YOU EAT

I am going to ask you to do something difficult. I am going to ask you to change how you eat, to embrace a healthy diet. I must warn you that a healthy diet requires commitment, a commitment that is especially difficult in a world filled with unhealthy temptations.

I also want you to be patient. Please don't try to change your life overnight. Too often people walk out of my office determined to do the right thing and desperate to make the changes as fast as they can, and they end up failing. Remember, it took you a long time to get where you are, and it will take time for you to change. If you try to change overnight, you'll only end up feeling miserable the next day, missing all those things you once enjoyed. This is why diets and New Year's reso-lutions fail. Permanent change occurs gradually, allowing you time to adjust.

I would be very happy if you dedicated yourself to making and sticking to one healthy change every week. For instance, next week start to eat fish every Monday night. The next week, in addi-tion to Monday night fish, start exercising every Wednesday morning. Then the next week, in addi-tion to Monday fish and Wednesday exercise, start Saturday by breakfasting on a high-fiber cereal with fresh fruit. Get the idea? This way, you make the changes gradually so they become a part of your everyday life.

Too many people confuse diet with weight loss. What follows has nothing to do with weight loss. In fact, I rarely, if ever, talk about weight loss to my patients. Rather, I emphasize that if you eat a healthy diet and exercise, the weight loss will come by itself. The problem with concentrating on weight loss is that it fixates you on a goal—losing five, ten, or however many pounds. Do you know what happens to people who are strictly goal-oriented? Once they've met their goal and the weight is off, they forget about the diet and then, guess what, they pack those pounds right back on again. Weight loss forces people to think in the short term. Healthy living forces you to think about the rest of your life.

How can a healthy diet work for people with allergies? In addition to helping you avoid illness, healthy living can make your allergies either go away or become much more manageable. Even better, the advice you're about to read can help any condition. For instance, I have seen diabetes and hypertension disappear or improve dramatically through simple diet and weight loss. The same is true of allergies. Many people who read this book and follow its advice will either rid themselves of allergies or, at the very least, will make their allergies infinitely more tolerable. That said, let's jump right into diet and see what you should eat to beat allergies.

### Fruits and Vegetables 101: Carotenoids and Flavonoids

Remember when you were young and your mother made you eat your vegetables? Mom was on to something. Vegetables and fruits, especially the brightly colored ones, are rich in carotenoids and flavonoids. There are about 600 different carotenoids, but only fourteen of these fat-soluble compounds concern humans. For nutritionists, the most important carotenoids are alpha-carotene, beta-carotene, lutein, lycopene, and zeaxanthin. Besides being able to reduce allergy-related symptoms, carotenoids and flavonoids, potent antioxidants that are found in many fruits and vegetables, are believed to play important roles in preventing heart disease, cataracts, and macular degeneration.

For instance, one group of researchers from the University of Auckland, New Zealand, examined data from fifty-three nations that participated in the International Study of Asthma and Allergies in Childhood (ISAAC) and found there was "a consistent pattern of decreases in the symptoms of allergic rhinoconjunctivitis and atopic eczema that was associated with an increased per-capita consumption of calories from cereal and rice, protein from cereal, nuts, and starch, as well as vegetables and vegetable nutrients. If the average daily consumption of these foods increases, it is speculated that an important decrease in symptom prevalence may be achieved." Statements like this speak for themselves. Eat more grains and vegetables and your allergy symptoms will probably be reduced—simple as that!

## Flavonoids: Quercetin

Flavonoids, water-soluble pigments found in plants, are important antioxidants and aid in the absorption of vitamin C. Flavonoids also possess a variety of antiallergic, antihistamine, anti-inflammatory, antioxidant, antiviral, and antimast cell activity that is related to their ability to modify arachidonic acid metabolism. Popular flavonoids include quercetin, found in onions, and genistein, commonly found in soy. Flavonoids can also be found in apples, cit-

**Antihistamine**
*Generic term for any agent that blocks the release or action of histamine.*

rus fruits, wine, and tea, and are often major components of an herb's therapeutic activity.

Natural quercetin boasts a variety of anti-inflammatory, antihistamine, antioxidant, antineutrophil, and anticancer effects. Found in apples, beans, green and black tea, many herbs, leafy green vegetables, and onions, quercetin is used in the treatment of allergies, arteriosclerosis, asthma, capillary disorders, and diabetes. Quercetin exerts its anti-allergy effects by inhibiting leukotriene and histamine release. Leukotrienes and histamine are major contributors to the series of sequential interactions known as the allergy cascade.

Several animal studies have found that this flavonoid can block histamine-mediated anaphylaxis. There is considerable empirical evidence that quercetin plays a role in allergy therapy, but to date there have only been two human studies examining the impact of quercetin on allergies. A Japanese study found that quercetin was at times almost *twice* as effective as the allergy drug sodium cromoglycate at preventing histamine release from mast cells in individuals with allergic rhinitis. Another study, from Russia, reported that "quercetin was found to be useful for the treatment of children with pollinosis." Both studies, published in 1995 in the *Journal of Allergy and Immunology,* show that further investigation is warranted, given the fact that histamine is a major contributor to the allergic reaction.

**Arachidonic Acid**
*The basic chemical unit from which inflammatory and allergic mediators like prostaglandin and leukotrienes are derived.*

## Dosages:

**Flavonoids:** Do as your mother told you and eat your fruits and vegetables. Several different flavonoid supplements are available, and the rec-

ommended dosage is 1,000 mg of citrus flavonoids daily.

**Quercetin:** For people with allergies, the standard
quercetin dose is 400 mg two to three times a day,
taken five to ten minutes before a meal.

## More Reasons to Eat Your Fruits and Vegetables

While fruits and vegetables contain all those allergy-friendly carotenoids and flavonoids, the story
only begins there. These same fruits and vegetables are packed with a whole slew of vital nutrients, such as vitamins A, C, and E that can, as we
will learn in Chapter 5, play a role in the treatment
of allergies.

## Meat versus Fish

What if I told you that you can have your meat and
eat it, too? There's nothing wrong with a little
meat, I just want you to eat more fish and less
meat. And while I'm talking about meat versus
fish, I want to briefly mention fat. There is good fat
and bad fat. Meat fat tends to be bad fat, whereas fish fat is usually good fat. The same caveat
goes for meat: not all meats are created equal.
There is little question that meat contains vital
proteins and nutrients, but chicken and game
meats are healthier than T-bone steaks and spare
ribs. If you can't live without red meat, however,
consider such naturally lean meats as ostrich and
venison that pack a low-fat, high-nutrition punch.
And, adding barbecue or steak sauce to them will
do wonders to improve the flavor of these low-fat
game meats.

If you can't find game meat at your grocery
store, ask your grocer where to get some. If there
are no suppliers in your area, there are several
online retailers that can ship you all the game

meat you want. If you insist on beef, or similar high-fat meat, try to buy the lean cuts and have the excess fat trimmed.

And every time you sink your teeth into a piece of meat, think about the study from Taiwan which found that teenagers who ate "butcher's meat" or liver had over 1.5 times the risk of asthma. You may not have asthma, but asthma and allergies do often go together, and what increases the risk of one frequently increases the risk of the other. Take, for instance, the 2001 study in the journal *Clinical and Experimental Allergy* which found that the risk of allergic rhinitis increased with liver consumption.

## Omega-3 and Omega-6— Essential Fatty Acids (EFAs)

Just like meat, not all fats are created equal. Polyunsaturated fatty acids, such as omega-3 and omega-6, are what we call good fats, whereas the saturated fats that are commonly found in baked goods—donuts and potato chips, for example— are bad fats. The best thing about fish is that it is rich in omega-3-fatty acids, a fat that may help you live longer. One Harvard study examined the dietary habits of 84,688 adults and found that people who ate fish two to four times a week slashed their risk of heart disease by 31 percent. And related benefits have been reported in study after study.

There is also evidence that a high intake of fish can protect against allergies. One Italian study found that 3 grams of fish-oil concentrate a day for thirty days improved lung function in people with seasonal allergic asthma. Specifically, airway con-striction was 265 percent prior to supplementation with fish oil, a number that plummeted to 37 per-cent after supplementation.

Considering the important role that fish oils

play in preserving overall health, eating fish can only help. Fish work their magic through the essential fatty acids (fish oils) like omega-3 and omega-6. The chief omega-3 fatty acids are eicos- apentaenoic acid (EPA) and docosahexaenoic acid (DHA), which can be found in deepwater fish, such as albacore tuna, anchovies, herring, salmon, and sardines. You can also find omega-3 in flaxseed oil, walnut oil, and game meat. For a really heavy intake of DHA and EPA, try the old favorite, cod liver oil, which has been greatly modified to get rid of its former offensively fishy taste.

For eczema sufferers, there is evidence that fish oils can help relieve their symptoms through its ability to reduce leukotriene-B4 production, a chemical mediator believed to be partially re- sponsible for eczema. In a double-blind, placebo- controlled, twelve-week clinical trial, researchers gave 1.8 grams of EPA in 10 grams of fish oil to a group of people with atopic dermatitis. The other group received no fish oil. After the twelve weeks, the fish-oil group had a significant reduction in itching, scaling, and "overall subjective severity" as compared to the placebo group.

**Atopic Dermatitis**

*Also known as eczema, this is a skin lesion that directly results from atopy, and is characterized by itching, scaling, and redness.*

While omega-6 is a good fat, an unbalanced amount of it may increase your risk of heart disease and high blood pressure. Another reason why you don't want to go overboard on omega-6 is because some experts suspect that excess omega-6 may actually make your allergies worse. Authorities hypothesize that our increased consumption of omega-6, coupled with our de - creased intake of omega-3, is in part responsible for the rising incidence of allergies. Omega-6 is under suspicion because it is used to make arachi- donic acid that, in turn, can be converted to

**Prostaglandins**
Substances that are involved in a wide range of body functions. Inflammatory in nature, they can cause airway constriction and increased blood flow.

prostaglandin E2 (PGE2) and leukotrienes, two major players in the allergy cascade. Even worse, PGE2 can, in turn, increase the production of IgE. Conversely, EPA and DHA are known to inhibit PGE2 and leukotriene synthesis, which is beneficial to allergic individuals. I strongly recommend that you maintain a healthy balance between the two omegas, since these fats are essential and your body must have them.

## Dosage

**Fish Oils:** The standard recommendation is 10 grams of fish oil a day. Some recommend supplements with a ratio of four times the amount of omega-3s to omega-6s because the normal American diet contains an unbalanced amount of omega-6s. You can meet these requirements simply by mixing a tablespoon of flaxseed oil with your favorite food daily. It is also a good idea to accompany the fish-oil supplementation with an antioxidant like vitamin E to preserve the potency of these oils because they are extremely sensitive to oxygen degradation. If you prefer not to take supplements, keep in mind that oily fish like salmon or sardines are rich in essential fatty acids.

## Meat versus No Meat

There is something to be said for not eating meat, not only on philosophical grounds, but even more important for our purposes, because a vegetarian diet is clearly a healthy diet. After reviewing the literature on diet and allergy, and taking into consideration the vital role that fruits and vegetables play, I strongly recommend a vegetarian diet to anyone who can tolerate it. At best, a vegetarian diet will help your allergies. At worst, a vegetarian diet will not help your allergies, but you'll probably end up living a longer, healthier life. As with eating fish, you can't lose by being a vegetarian.

The truth about vegetarianism, however, is that not everyone, myself included, can live without meat, fish, and dairy products. I strike a balance by rarely eating meat, and having most of my evening meals consist of fish. I do try to eat a vegetarian breakfast and lunch when possible. For those of you who believe vegetarianism is the best path, just remember to supplement your diet with calcium, iron, selenium, vitamin $B_{12}$, vitamin D, and zinc, because a diet without meat, fish, or dairy products can translate into several vitamin/ mineral deficiencies. You should also consider a daily multivitamin/mineral because it will help prevent these deficiencies.

# CHAPTER 5

# ALLERGY-FRIENDLY SUPPLEMENTS

**M**any people turn to natural remedies because they are not satisfied with traditional Western approaches. One study reported that a mere 26 percent of people with allergies believed that their symptoms were well controlled, with another 52 percent believing that therapies existed that actually worked. Given these considerations, it is not surprising that integrative medicine has exploded over the past three decades. I'm one of these type-A personality New York City doctors who was raised by big, stodgy, academic medical centers that fed me a steady diet of conventional Western medicine. If I didn't know that tobacco and alcohol were bad, I'd probably be like Winston Churchill, sitting in some dark, smoky back room with a very large cigar in one hand and a glass of Scotch in the other, growling with disdain at anything that even hinted of integrative medicine.

I'm here to tell you that even old-school New York City doctors can turn a new leaf. When I started writing about integrative medicine six years ago, I was skeptical about vitamins, minerals, herbs, and any other therapy that didn't involve high technology or at least a powerful pharmaceutical with lots of juicy side effects. As I researched my articles, it slowly dawned on me that some of it really works. I was pleasantly surprised to learn that the people who perform this research come from similar backgrounds and suffer the same trials and tribulations every scientist faces when seeking that elusive thing called truth. Although I am still learning, it has forever changed the way I look at health and medicine. So, before we delve into supplements for allergies, let us briefly examine the problems scientists and physicians face when conducting such research.

## The Challenges of Nutritional Research

Vitamin deficiencies usually occur in one of three ways in humans: inadequate intake, improper absorption, or increased demand. Investigators have conducted research into vitamin/mineral supplements to determine if replacing a specific deficiency can improve or eliminate allergies. One of the problems associated with supplement research is that, if an individual is deficient in one substance, chances are she or he is also deficient in other substances. Vitamin and mineral deficiencies do not occur in a vacuum, since the dietary or medical problems that created the deficiency usually cause other deficiencies. Knowing this, you can see why it is difficult to study one partic-ular deficiency without taking others into consid-eration. Then, when you have five or six different deficiencies, you can see how research rapidly becomes complicated.

The second challenge facing supplement research is that proper immune function does not rest on a single nutrient, but on an entire symphony of vitamins and minerals that are responsible for overall health. This is why it is so difficult to test the impact of specific vitamin/mineral supplementation on allergies.

As you read this chapter, you will notice most researchers report that a particular supplement benefited some, but not all, study participants.

For example, in a study examining the effect of a particular supplement on allergies, the authors may report that only 54 percent of the participants had a favorable response to supplements. This is a common finding because the medical condition we call allergies is the result of many different pathways. Many roads lead to allergies and each individual has a unique set of genetic and environmental influences that result in the expression of some, but not all, of these pathways.

These unique pathways are the reason why we have multiple types of allergies that often respond to different treatment. Variety may be the spice of life, but these many pathways present a special challenge to researchers since we are still in the process of understanding how they work and interact. Allergies clearly result from a complex interplay between genes and the environment, and this is why we see a particular supplement work for some, but not all, people. The good news is, as our knowledge grows, we are beginning to understand that, while many roads lead to allergies, they all tend to end at the same place, and some of our most successful therapies target these common pathways.

Researchers also have to contend with different diets among the study subjects. The ideal supplement study would examine two groups of identical people with identical medical conditions, nutrient deficiencies, and diets while comparing the effect of supplementation versus no supplementation. Although it is relatively easy to find people with similar medical conditions, it is difficult to control and fully monitor individual diets. With animal studies, you can totally control an animal's diet. That means all gerbils get the same number of grams of the same food each and every day, and only one group receives the supplement. The other tough part about diets and research studies is that people cheat—a lot! Scientists do have mathematical models that correct data for different diets, but dietary aberrations will always remain a potential source of confusion and error.

## So What Are You Going to Do?

As with any emerging field of medicine, some controversy exists over the true impact that supplements have on allergies. Nevertheless, despite the complexities of nutrient research, there is a substantial body of literature indicating that, for many people with allergies, there are supplements that can help. Given the number of potential supplements, it's natural to wonder, "How do I choose the supplements that are right for me?" Since nobody wants to be popping fifty pills a day, let me help you figure this out.

Being an old-school physician, I used to believe there was no substitute for a healthy diet and that supplements were, at best, a second line of defense. I still believe there is no substitute for a healthy diet, coupled with adequate sleep and exercise, but in this increasingly toxic world, I have reconsidered my position on nutritional supplements. Our increasingly toxic environment routinely delivers an excessive oxidant load that frequently overwhelms the antioxidant defenses of our bodies. Given these considerations, I strongly recommended that every person with allergies supplement their diets with one or two antioxidants, in addition to a healthy diet, regular exercise, and adequate sleep.

My personal favorites are vitamin C and a multivitamin. I suggest you choose one or two standard supplements that are tailored to your individual needs. If, for instance, your family has a history of heart disease and high cholesterol, vitamin C would be a great choice as a standard dietary supplement, since it is a major antioxidant and studies have shown that ascorbic acid reduces choles-terol. One study of more than 6,000 adults found that those with the highest levels of vitamin C had an impressive 27-percent reduction in heart dis-ease and a 26-percent lower incidence of stroke.

What I'd like you to do is start taking two stan-dard supplements that will not only help your allergies, but will also protect you against the dis-eases you may personally be at risk for. Your aller-gies will probably improve after one to two months of taking these supplements. After two months, if your symptoms are still not reduced as much as you'd like, I suggest you continue taking your two standard antioxidants and experiment with additional individual supplements to see which vitamin or mineral offers your allergies the most relief. Give each supplement a four-week trial while recording your symptoms in your allergy diary. You might also want to get tested for vitamin and mineral deficiencies and correct any defici-ency found.

I also want you to remember that nutritional supplements can help people with allergies, but they are only one piece of the complex puzzle we call health. The foundation of a healthy life also demands a clean environment, good nutrition, regular exercise, and adequate sleep, and the whole purpose of this book is to use an entire range of procedures to eliminate or markedly improve your allergies. That said, here are some of the supplements that can potentially help alleviate your symptoms and make your life better.

## Borage Oil

Derived from a pretty blue star-shaped plant called *Borago officinalis*, the herbal supplement borage oil is rich in gamma linolenic acid (GLA). In the body, GLA is converted to prostaglandin E1 (PGE1), a potent anti-inflammatory and immune-system regulator that can help in the treatment of allergic eczema.

Studies have demonstrated that adults and infants with eczema and other dermatological disorders are often deficient in GLA due to an abnormality in fatty acid metabolism, and several studies report that borage oil can help people with eczema. One Italian study of twenty-four people found that supplementing with borage oil for four to eight weeks caused a "significant reduction in inflammation, dryness, scaliness, and itch—without side effects" in patients with atopic dermatitis. Another Swedish study examined the effects of borage oil on infantile seborrheic dermatitis (diaper rash) in forty-eight children and reported that, after twelve days of treatment, "all the children were free from skin lesions, even in the areas not treated with the oil." According to the authors of the study, when the treatment was discontinued, the lesions reappeared, but "with intermittent therapy two to three times a week, there were no recurrences." In this study, the children were treated until six to seven months of age, after which the treatment was successfully discontinued.

**Dosage:** Borage seed oil contains approximately 20 to 26 percent GLA. Take according to label instructions. For topical administration, 0.5 milliliters of oil is applied to the diaper area daily for fourteen days, then two to three times weekly once the rash disappears. No serious side effects or drug interactions are reported. Avoid any borage-oil preparation that contains pyrrolizidine, alkaloids, a potential liver toxin.

## Bromelain

Believe it or not, this substance, derived from pineapple plants, may help people with allergies.

As an established mucolytic agent, it helps break down thick mucous secretions, and it also acts as an anti-inflammatory by inhibiting the synthesis of prostaglandin and arachidonic acid. To date, there have been no clinical studies that examine bromelain's role in relieving allergic symptoms.

> **Mucolytic**
> *Generic term for a substance that can break down mucous and make it thinner. These substances are often used to treat allergy symptoms.*

**Dosage:** 400–500 mg three times a day on an empty stomach. If you are allergic to pineapples, you should not use bromelain. Drug interactions are reported with amoxicillin, coumadin, erythromycin, penicillamine, penicillin V, and warfarin. If you are using any of these medications, talk to a doctor knowledgeable about their interaction with bromelain before taking the bromelain.

## Evening Primrose Oil

Like its cousin borage oil, evening primrose oil is rich in gamma linolenic acid (GLA), which is converted in the body to prostaglandin E1, a powerful anti-inflammatory. Used in the treatment of diabetes and rheumatoid arthritis, there is also evidence that GLA may have anticancer activity.

Research has shown that people with eczema are often deficient in gamma-linolenic acid due to a defect in fatty-acid metabolism. Several studies have found that GLA-rich evening primrose oil (EPO) can help people with eczema. One double-blind, placebo-controlled study published in *The Lancet* examined the impact of EPO in ninety-nine patients with atopic eczema and reported "a significant clinical improvement—[with] no side effects." According to the authors of the study, the subjects reported decreased itch, scaling, and redness after using the oil. Another double-blind, randomized, placebo-controlled British trial demonstrated similar results in children and adults, reporting a "significant improvement." Finally, a Finnish double-blind, placebo-controlled study found that after twelve weeks of EPO treatment in patients with atopic eczema, there was a "statistically significant improvement—in the percentage of the body surface involved by eczema as well as in dryness and itch—[with] a significant reduction in inflammation."

**Dosage:** Most studies use a daily dose of 6,000 mg of EPO that contains 570 mg of GLA. No significant side effects or drug interactions are reported with EPO. It is also a good idea to add a multivitamin/mineral containing magnesium, niacin, zinc, and vitamins C and $B_6$, as these nutrients are also needed to make prostaglandin E1.

## Vitamin A (Retinol)

I hope this section enlightens you to the benefits of vitamin A, especially if you're reading this at night since, without retinol, you will not be able to see the light. Vitamin A helps with retinol deficiency that can result in night blindness. Vitamin A also helps to keep the epithelial cells that line our airways healthy, a vital line of defense against bacteria and viruses. Besides helping to protect against infection, vitamin A stimulates immune function and has an anti-inflammatory action.

Vitamin A is found in dairy products, fruits, liver, meats, poultry, vegetables, and cod liver oil. Beta-carotene, a powerful antioxidant carotenoid found in fruits and vegetables, can be converted by the body into vitamin A. Despite being a relatively weak antioxidant, vitamin A is used to treat a number of conditions, including acne, celiac disease, measles, and night blindness.

An association between increased vitamin A intake and a reduced risk of airway disease has been demonstrated, and a deficiency of vitamin A has a detrimental effect on the airways. Animal studies have also shown that vitamin A deficiency can increase airway constriction, a potentially major problem for people with allergic asthma. Adding insult to injury, it appears that a vitamin A deficiency also increases the inflammatory response, a finding echoed by a Swedish study which reported that vitamin A–deficient rodents had elevated mast cell levels, increased skin reactions to histamine, and they "displayed a consistently stronger immediate skin reaction" following antigen injection.

This association between vitamin A deficiency and airway disease was supported in a paper in the *American Review of Respiratory Disease*. Researchers at Johns Hopkins examined data from more than 3,800 people who participated in the National Health and Nutrition Examination Survey (NHANES I) and concluded "that a diet poor in vitamin A increases the risk of airway obstruction." While the NHANES I study was primarily concerned with asthma, evidence that vitamin A can help people with allergies is found in a 2001 issue of *International Archives of Allergy and Immunology*, which reported that retinol inhibits eosinophils and basophils. Further supporting vitamin A in fighting allergic disease was one German study that found that retinoids could limit IgE production, an effect that was particularly prominent in patients with atopic dermatitis. Studies examining whether or not

**Eosinophil**
*One of several immune system cells that can release histamine during an allergic reaction. Eosinophils can also kill invading bacteria.*

**Basophil**
*Similar to the mast cells, basophils are one of several immune-system cells that participate in allergic reactions. They are chiefly responsible for releasing histamine.*

vitamin A can actually reduce allergic symptoms (sneezing and runny nose, for example) are still pending.

**Dosage:** 10,000–25,000 IU of vitamin A daily is recommended for long-term supplementation. Vitamin A is best absorbed when taken with food.

**Side Effects:** Interactions have been described with cancer chemotherapy drugs, cholesterol-lowering drugs, and oral contraceptives. If you are using any of these medications, talk to a doctor knowledgeable about the interactions between drugs and supplements before taking vitamin A.

## Vitamin B$_6$ (Pyridoxine)

Pyridoxine plays a critical role in the manufacture and breakdown of amino acids, the building blocks of proteins and hormones. Along with vitamin B$_{12}$ and folic acid, vitamin B$_6$ lowers homocysteine levels. A by-product of protein metabolism, elevated homocysteine has been identified as a risk factor for heart disease. Foods rich in vitamin B$_6$ include bananas, lentils, liver, potatoes, raisin bran, tuna, and turkey. Pyridoxine is used in the treatment of several conditions, including acne, celiac disease, depression, diabetes, and premenstrual syndrome.

As for the relationship between vitamin B$_6$ and allergies, one 1981 study reported that vitamin B$_6$ blocked histamine release from mast cells. As with most vitamin, mineral, and herbal research on allergies, trials examining the impact of B$_6$ supplements on allergies are limited. In fact, there is only one 1992 Russian study which found that "bronchial asthma and atopic dermatitis were treated more effectively" with maximal doses of B$_6$.

**Dosage:** 25–100 mg of vitamin B$_6$ once a day is recommended.

**Side Effects:** Do not take vitamin $B_6$ if you are using levodopa to treat Parkinson's disease. Rare side effects include fatigue, headache, and nausea. Interactions with antiseizure medications, barbiturates, and tricyclic antidepressants have been reported with vitamin $B_6$. If you are using any of these medications, talk to a doctor knowledgeable about the interactions between drugs and supplements before taking vitamin $B_6$.

## Vitamin C (Ascorbate, Ascorbic Acid)

Pound for pound, vitamin C is one of the most important vitamins when it comes to allergies. Not only is vitamin C the most powerful water-soluble free-radical scavenger (antioxidant), vitamin C also protects the heart by preventing LDL cholesterol oxidation. Antioxidants are crucial for people with allergies because increased oxidative stress has been implicated in several allergic diseases like asthma and atopic dermatitis. If you're sick of being sick, vitamin C in doses of 1–3 grams a day can shorten common cold symptoms by 23 percent. Besides scavenging free radicals, vitamin C plays a role in regenerating vitamin E, another powerful antioxidant. Found in many fruits and vegetables, vitamin C is especially abundant in broccoli, Brussels sprouts, citrus fruits, currants, kiwifruit, parsley, red peppers, rose hips, and strawberries.

Vitamin C also appears to play a pivotal role in allergies. In fact, research indicates that a vitamin-C deficiency can result in an exponential rise in histamine. There is a significant body of literature indicating that vitamin C can help people with allergies. One 1992 study from Arizona State University published in the *Journal of American Dietary Association* showed that vitamin C supplements reduce blood histamine levels by up to 40 percent.

Equally important, there is evidence indicating that vitamin C reduces IgE levels. As you may recall, IgE is the prime mediator of the allergic response, and elevated IgE levels are believed to correspond to allergy severity. Ready for more good news? According to a 2000 report published in *The Lancet*, researchers discovered that increased vitamin C intake reduces the risk of atopy, a major risk factor for asthma and allergies.

Scientists first began to discover that vitamin C can help people with allergies about sixty years ago. Studies in the 1940s indicated that vitamin C levels could be lowered "during hay-fever attacks" and that supplements helped allergic people. One pioneering work published in the journal *Science* in 1942 reported results ranging from "great relief" to "almost no hay fever" after 200–500 mg of daily ascorbic acid. More recent work includes a 1973 study by Yale scientists, which found that pretreating with vitamin C reduced histamine-induced constriction of the airways. In 1990, Italian researchers found that 2 grams of vitamin C "significantly" inhibited the effect of histamine on the airways in people with allergic rhinitis.

A 1991 study examined the effect of intranasal vitamin C in allergic rhinitis in sixty people who were divided into placebo and ascorbic-acid groups. According to the authors, "at two weeks, 74 percent of the patients treated with ascorbic acid solution were found to have lessened nasal edema, mucous secretion, and nasal blockage" as compared to only 24 percent of the placebo group. These researchers further reported that "a complete improvement occurred in nine patients and partial improvement in twelve." Of all the vitamin supplements, ascorbic acid boasts the most solid foundation of research supporting its role as a potent allergy fighter and supplementing with it is highly recommended for anyone with allergies.

**Dosage:** Most people take 1,000–3,000 mg of vitamin C a day divided between two and three doses.

**Side Effects:** While many people can tolerate 2,000–4,000 mg of vitamin C a day, doses above 2,000 mg a day can cause diarrhea. Other side effects include headache, heartburn, and vomiting. Interactions with acetaminophen (Tylenol), antibiotics, and warfarin have been reported with vitamin C. If you are using any of these medications, talk to a healthcare professional who is knowledgeable about the interactions between drugs and supplements before taking vitamin C.

## Vitamin E (Alpha-Tocopherol, Tocopherol)

Vitamin E is a generic term that includes eight fat-soluble molecules, only one of which, alpha-tocopherol, is active in humans. The body's leading lipid soluble antioxidant, vitamin E helps protect every organ and cell in our bodies from free-radical damage. There is a substantive body of evidence indicating that vitamin E protects against cancer, cataracts, diabetes, heart disease, high cholesterol, and macular degeneration. Though a super antioxidant, vitamin E can't do the job alone and interacts synergistically with beta-carotene, selenium, vitamin C, and a host of other nutrients to protect our bodies from free radicals.

Being a fat-soluble vitamin, it is not surprising that natural alpha-tocopherol is found in fatty foods, such as egg yolks, nuts and seeds, and almond, sunflower, and wheat germ vegetable oils. Mercifully for your cholesterol, whole-grain cereals and leafy green vegetables are also good tocopherol sources.

There is strong evidence that vitamin E limits the allergic response. IgE is a major allergy mediator, and people with asthma and allergies often have elevated IgE in their blood. Harvard and the University of Nottingham conducted a collaborative study on 2,633 adults that examined the effect of vitamin E on IgE. This study, published in a 2000 issue of *The Lancet,* concluded that, "higher concentrations of vitamin E intake were associated with lower serum IgE concentrations and a lower frequency of allergen sensitization." The study also found that increased vitamin E intake reduced "airway hyper-responsiveness, hayfever, and asthma."

**Neutrophils**
*A mature leucocyte (white blood cell) that plays a central role in many inflammatory reactions. Neutrophils also kill invading organisms.*

How does vitamin E work its magic? Evidence suggests that vitamin E blocks the activation of neutrophils, which are potent inflammatory cells. Along with vitamin C, vitamin E supplements get a strong thumbs-up for anyone with allergies.

**Dosage:** 400–800 IU daily. Natural vitamin E is the preferred form. When reading a vitamin E label, a "d" before the name "alpha-tocopherol" means the supplement is from a natural source. If you see a "dl" before the "alpha-tocopherol" it means the supplement is synthetic. Synthetic vitamin E only comes in the alpha form, whereas natural vitamin E also comes in the alpha form but can be mixed with the also beneficial beta, delta, and gamma forms. And just when you thought vitamin E could not get any more confusing, d-alpha-tocopherol comes in acetate and succinate forms that differ slightly in potency. But all you really need to know is that *natural* vitamin E is more active and better absorbed than its synthetic counterpart and is the preferred supplement. Remember that d=natural whereas dl=synthetic.

**Side Effects:** Side effects are rare and are usually seen with prolonged dosages over 1,000 IU a day. Potential side effects include abdominal pain, diarrhea, and headache. Drug interactions have been reported with aspirin, coumadin, and glyburide. If you are using any of these medications, speak to a doctor knowledgeable about the interactions between drugs and supplements before adding vitamin E to your supplement list.

Vitamin E should not be taken with alcohol or iron pills, since alcohol decreases absorption and inorganic iron destroys vitamin E.

## Selenium

King of the antioxidant minerals, selenium works synergistically with vitamin E to protect our hearts and lungs from disease. Selenium is also a cancer fighter through its activation of glutathione peroxidase, a potent antioxidant enzyme. A study published in the *Journal of the American Medical Association* reported that people who took 200 mcg of yeast-based selenium for an average of four and a half years had a 50 percent reduction in overall cancer risk. Especially important for people with allergies, selenium is vital for a healthy immune system. Used for cancer prevention and heart disease, the most important natural sources of selenium are Brazil nuts, grains, organ meats, plant products, seafood, and yeast.

Not surprisingly, a selenium deficiency is found in people with allergic asthma and food allergies. Animal studies have found that selenium can help block a variety of allergic reactions. One Russian study found that selenium-enriched baker's yeast blocked anaphylactic food allergy in rodents.

A Korean study found that pretreatment with selenium inhibited allergy-induced asthma in the lungs of laboratory mice. While there exists an extensive body of literature documenting the antioxidant and anti-inflammatory actions of selenium, human studies on selenium and allergies are still lacking. Nevertheless, preliminary research is encouraging.

**Dosage:** 200 mcg a day is the recommended amount.

**Side Effects:** Side effects, such as selenosis, usually occur with doses over 600 mcg a day. Selenosis is characterized by dry hair, fatigue, and irritability. Drug interactions have been reported with cisplatin, clozapine, and valproic acid. If you are using any of these medications, speak to a healthcare professional who is knowledgeable about the interactions between drugs and supplements before taking selenium.

## Thymus Gland Extract (Thymomodulin)

The thymus gland is located in the lower part of the neck and is intimately involved in immune function. The two basic types of immune response are antibody mediated (as in vaccinations) and cell mediated (as in the immune-system cells themselves—the primary ones being the natural killer cells, the T cells, and the suppressor cells). Cell-mediated immunity plays a critical role in protecting our bodies against disease caused by bacteria, parasites, yeast, and viruses. Cell-mediated immunity also helps protect against allergies and this is where the thymus gland steps in, being the chief regulator of cell-mediated immunity. Thymus gland extracts are commercially available and are used to treat a variety of ailments including the common cold and asthma. The reason given for the success of these extracts is that they restore proper immune function.

One Italian study examined the impact of 120 mg of daily thymomodulin for four months on twenty people with allergic rhinitis. According to the study's authors, thymomodulin "significantly reduced" the number of "allergic episodes" with a reduction of symptoms and a "normalization of IgE." Further testimony to thymomodulin's abilities came from a 1989 study which found that thymomodulin "significantly reduced" airway responsiveness to methacholine, an airway constrictor, in patients with allergic asthma.

Another study compared an exclusion diet to one combined with thymomodulin for the prevention of food allergies in children. Researchers divided forty-four children into two groups. Group A had only an exclusion diet, and group B had thymomodulin combined with the exclusion diet. After several months, the scientists performed a food challenge. (A food challenge involves the ingestion of increasing doses of the suspected allergy-provoking food while the person is being monitored for allergy symptoms. The test is usually performed in the fasting state, with the test subject having refrained from eating that particular food for one to two weeks prior to the challenge. Given the potential for severe allergic reaction, food challenges are normally performed in a hospital or clinic setting.) Only 29 percent of the group-B children experienced a relapse, compared to 68 percent in the group-A children. As with other studies, the authors reported a "significant decrease" in IgE.

Finally, another Italian double-blind, controlled clinical trial examined the effect of a food challenge on nineteen children with atopic dermatitis related to food allergies who had been given either a placebo or thymomodulin. According to the authors, after two weeks, the thymomodulin-treated group had no change in their skin lesions, whereas the placebo group had a worsening of their symptoms.

**Dosage:** Thymomodulin is not presently available in the United States, but a variety of other thymus gland extracts are. Dosage depends on the manufacture's directions. No significant side effects are reported with the use of thymus gland extract.

# CHAPTER 6

# HERBS AND OTHER ALTERNATIVE THERAPIES

Through millions of years of trial and error, civilization has found that certain plants have medicinal properties, and for millennia they have traditionally been used, with effectiveness, as healing therapies. Recently, with the emergence of modern chemistry, pharmaceutical companies have been able to isolate and synthesize the magic our ancestors discovered, sometimes enhancing their therapeutic benefits and eliminating side effects. There is always the danger, though, that using only part of an herb will diminish its time-tested effectiveness, and there is the further problem that this synthesis can result in toxic waste products harmful to the environment.

There are, and probably will always be, problems with the way pharmaceuticals are made and marketed. The pharmaceutical industry is far from perfect, and drug-related illnesses and deaths are far too common. The April 15, 1998 issue of the *Journal of the American Medical Association* (*JAMA*) reports 106,000 deaths in one year (1994) from drug reactions, and this number is probably underestimated. On the plus side, there are people walking this Earth who might not be here today without them. Stop and think for a moment about all the people who might have died were it not for antibiotics, cancer drugs, or heart medications.

The same can be said of the herbal industry. Integrative therapies and their associated products represent a multibillion dollar industry that rivals the pharmaceutical industry. Like pharmaceutical companies, the herbal industry has its strengths and weaknesses, but unlike drugs, herbs are usually far less likely to have life-threatening side effects. Medicinal herbs frequently offer consumers products that are not available elsewhere, and standardized herbal products manufactured by reputable companies are usually preservative- and additive-free, an important consideration for people with allergies.

One of the greatest challenges faced by the herbal industry is standardization, and, with some preparations, a consumer can never really be sure how much active ingredient they are taking, although the most reputable brands have standardized active ingredients and always list them on the label. While pharmaceuticals may be standardized across the board, their downside is that they often contain preservatives and food colorings, which can spell trouble for people with allergies, a problem rarely seen with natural products. The vast majority of herbal manufacturers are responsible, and the number of adulterated and mislabeled herbal products that still manage to find their way to the market are few and far between. As for efficacy, we are beginning to see serious, rigorous studies on herbal products published in respected journals like the *Journal of the American Medical Association*. While these publications are encouraging, herbal research is still in its infancy and documenting efficacy often takes years of research and controversy.

Finally, while pharmaceutical companies can have a devastating impact on the environment, so too can herbs. Take, for instance, the herb goldenseal (*Hydrastis canadensis*); it is becoming endangered because of its medicinal properties. Again, there are two sides to every story. The herbal industry may not be perfect, but if it were not for botanicals that have been used for thousands and thousands of years, many of the people walking this Earth would not be here today. Stop and think for a moment about all the lives herbs have saved through the millennia.

This is the approach to integrative/complementary and conventional Western medicine I hope to share with you. I want you to appreciate all their strengths and weaknesses. Like vitamins, minerals, and pharmaceuticals, the herb that works for your friend may not work for you.

Herbs can help people with allergies, and, as with vitamin and mineral supplements, combined herbal formulations tend to work better than solitary agents, a phenomenon herbalists call "orchestration," or "creating a symphony." Remember that many of our most powerful drugs had a humble start as a "weed" in somebody's backyard.

### *Avena sativa* (Oats)

This herb not only relieves the itch of eczema, but also can help lower your triglyceride levels. An oatmeal bath is reported to help relieve hives and itchy skin. You can make an oatmeal bath by running water through a cheesecloth that contains several tablespoons of oats.

### *Ephedra sinica* (Ephedrine, Ma Huang, Desert Herb, Desert Tea, and Mormon Tea)

A Chinese shrub that has been used for more than 5,000 years, *Ephedra sinica* is a natural source of ephedrine, a common ingredient in asthma, allergy, and cough preparations. While the ephedra shrub is found in many desert climates, it is the Asian species that is medicinally active through the alkaloids ephedrine and pseudoephedrine.

For people with allergies, the chief benefits of ephedrine is its anti-inflammatory activity.

While the effects of pharmaceutical ephedrine on allergies are well known, research examining herbal ephedra in allergies is scant. One study from China reported that liquid Ma Huang lowered IgE levels. Synthetic ephedrine is available, but some authorities believe the herbal form may be safer for people with allergies because it is "better tolerated" and causes fewer side effects.

**Dosage:** Dosage varies according to preparation. Consult the manufacturer's instructions or a knowledgable healthcare professional for appropriate dosing. Chronic use of ephedra is not recommended.

**Side Effects:** Ephedra acts as a stimulant and, if abused, can have amphetamine-like side effects, including a fast heart rate and palpitations. Do not use ephedra if you have diabetes or heart disease. Ephedra is potentially addictive, and, in high dosages, it can be poisonous and even lead to death, so caution is required.

Since ephedra can suppress adrenal gland function, you'll need to take magnesium, pantothenic acid, vitamin $B_6$, and vitamin C supplements if you intend to use it for an extended period of time. Pseudoephedrine can make you sleepy, so avoid driving or performing potentially hazardous activities like operating heavy machinery when using ephedra. *Ephedra sinica* must be protected from light.

### *Hamamelis virginiana* (Witch Hazel)

Found in North America and Europe, witch hazel is used to treat cold sores, canker sores, and hemorrhoids. Considered to have anti-inflammatory action, witch hazel creams have traditionally been used to treat allergic eczema. According to one double-blind trial, witch hazel applied four times daily was as effective as a prescription drug (bufexamac) in treating eczema.

**Dosage:** Apply to the affected area four times daily. There are no significant side effects or drug interactions associated with topical use.

### *Sambucus nigra* (Elderberry)

Found in both Europe and North America, the blue and black berries of the elderberry plant are most commonly used by herbalists to treat influenza. Being rich in flavonoids and quercetin, elderberry may help allergic people. To date, there are no studies that examine elderberry use in allergies.

**Flavonoid**
*Substance found in many plant products that has a variety of antioxidant and anti-inflammatory properties.*

**Dosage:** Black elderberry extract syrup: 5–15 milliliters for children, 10–30 milliliters in adults, twice daily. Similarly, an infusion may be prepared from brewing 3–4 grams of dried flowers in 150 milliliters of water for five minutes, then straining, and taking two to three times daily. Only use products that are made from the ripe elderberry or dried flowers, as the leaves, stems, roots, and unripe berries can cause nausea, vomiting, and diarrhea. No harmful drug interactions are reported with elderberry.

### *Tylophora asthmatica* (*Tylophora indica*, Indian Ipecac)

Native to Eastern and Southern India, tylophora has been used in the treatment of allergies and asthma. Tylophora's active ingredients are a pair of alkaloids that are reported to have anti-inflammatory, antihistamine and anti-mast-cell action. As you may recall, the mast cell is a major reservoir of histamine, the chemical that is most responsible for allergy symptoms.

Animal studies have found that tylophora can delay hypersensitivity and contact sensitivity. It is suspected that this immunosuppressive effect may result from the herb's ability to stimulate the adrenal glands to make natural steroids. One double-blind, placebo-controlled study of 110 individuals with asthma who consumed one tylophora leaf daily for six days reported that 62 percent of the tylophora group had "complete to moderate relief in symptoms of nasobronchial allergy" as compared to only 28 percent of the placebo group. The symptom relief lasted for up to twelve weeks.

**Dosage:** 200–400 mg of the dried herb daily, or 1–2 milliliters of 1:5 tincture for no more than two weeks. Do not use for more than four weeks at a time. There are no reported drug interactions, and the side effects, usually seen only with large doses, include nausea, oral pain, stomach upset, and vomiting.

## *Urtica dioica* (Nettle Leaf, Stinging Nettle)

Found in most temperate regions of the world, stinging nettle leaf can help people with allergies despite its stinging nature (nettle gets its stinging reputation from small hairs on the leaves that cause a burning sensation when in contact with skin). The leaves and roots of this plant have been used for centuries to treat conditions such as osteo-arthritis, coughing, and benign prostatic hyper - trophy. The active ingredients behind nettle's medicinal properties remain controversial, but it is believed that urtica acts as an anti-inflammatory. It is also theorized that the plant's histamine acts like a hormone to reduce the inflammatory response.

One randomized, double-blind study found

that 300 mg of freeze-dried nettle leaf help to relieve allergy symptoms. Fifty-eight percent of those who participated in the trial reported significant symptomatic relief, whereas 48 percent said *Urtica dioica* was "equally or more effective" than medications they had used. Reported to work well against grass allergies and classic hay fever, stinging nettle may help take the bite out of allergies.

**Dosage:** 300 mg two to three times a day, or 2–4 milliliters of tincture three times daily. The most common side effect is stomach upset, which can be prevented by taking nettle with food. Occasional skin rash has also been reported.

## Acupuncture

Although not an herbal remedy, acupuncture is a part of traditional Chinese medicine (TCM) and has been used for well over 2,000 years by the Chinese to treat virtually every medical condition known. Health, according to the Chinese, is determined by qi, the vital life energy that flows through every living thing, and acupuncture employs strategically placed needles in points along the meridians of the body to balance yin and yang and restore health by increasing this energy flow through channels. In one form of acupuncture, a small electric current is passed through the acupuncture needle to enhance this effect. While a complete discussion of this rich form of TCM is beyond the scope of this book, suffice it to say that there are about 671 specific acupuncture points with, some say, several thousand additional points located on the hands, head, and ears. In the West, acupuncture is primarily used to treat chronic pain and alcohol or drug abuse.

Acupuncture has also been used to treat allergies, and animal studies suggest that this ancient technique may produce an effect similar to steroids and suppress cellular immune function. One Chinese study examined the effect of electro-acupuncture in the treatment of allergic shock in mice and found that the mortality rate in the acupuncture group was only 26.7 percent as compared to 75 percent in the control group.

One study of twenty-two people with allergies demonstrated that acupuncture could help relieve allergy symptoms for two months following treatment. This study reported that 50 percent of the participants "were virtually symptom-free" at the end of the trial, with another 36 percent experiencing a "moderate reduction in symptoms." The authors also reported a drop in the "numbers of blood eosinophils" along with a 76-percent reduction in IgE levels.

## Hypnotherapy

Another alternative/complementary therapy, hypnosis has been used in the treatment of a variety of skin conditions, including acne, alopecia, atopic dermatitis, and vitiligo. One British study examined the effect of hypnosis in twenty children with "severe, resistant atopic dermatitis" and found that "all but one showed immediate improvement."

Even more impressive, at eighteen months, ten of the children "had maintained improvement in itching and scratching," and nine had shown less sleep disturbance. Similar results were reported by the same authors in eighteen adults with "extensive atopic dermatitis, resistant to conventional treatment."

# CHAPTER 7

# THE ROLE DRUGS PLAY IN ALLERGY RELIEF

**D**espite our best efforts, there will always be people who will need medication to control their allergic *symptoms*. Of all the allergy therapies discussed so far, allergy medicines have demonstrated that they are most helpful in reducing acute symptoms for the most people, if not in eliminating the allergies themselves.

Without question, the best offense is a good defense and source control coupled with ventilation is the most important intervention you can take when it comes to relief of allergy symptoms. Drugs can have dangerous side effects and are certainly not the best way to treat any medical condition, but, for some people, medications remain an occasional and, at times, a permanent fact of life.

There is no doubt that drugs can cause serious problems of their own and that antiallergy agents are notorious for side effects. While it is true that many medications can have deleterious side effects, and true that some physicians rely too heavily on medications to treat allergies, it is also true that there are millions of people whose lives have been improved by these agents.

Knowledge is power and the more you know about the medicines you take, the more effective they become. While the purpose of this book is to get you medication-free or dramatically reduce the amount of medication you are taking, the purpose of this chapter is to enlighten you about the side effects of allergy medications while extracting the most benefit. When used properly, drugs can be, symptom-wise at least, helpful, even if they do not cure the problem.

## Allergy Drugs

The distinguishing feature between traditional pharmacologic allergy management and complementary or naturopathic medicine is that allopathic Western medicine aims to block allergy symptoms and reduce inflammation, whereas the aim of naturopathic medicine is to limit immune system hyperreactivity while enhancing proper immune function. Traditionally, most antiallergy drugs fall into four categories that may be used alone or in combination. They are, antihistamines, decongestants, anticholinergics, and corticosteroids. While most of these agents, when used properly, can be safe and effective, some have a reputation for unpleasant and potentially lethal side effects, ranging from sedation to dangerous heart rhythms. For the majority of people with allergies, however, the most disturbing immediate side effects are the sedation and fatigue that can be particularly devastating when coupled with the sleep deprivation and cognitive dysfunction already caused by allergies.

## Antihistamines

Antihistamines do exactly what they sound like—they block H1 histamine receptors, thereby preventing allergy symptoms by interfering with the action of histamine. Antihistamines do an excellent job at relieving allergy symptoms and are the option of last resort when all else fails. The major problem with antihistamines is that the side effects can be worse than the allergies they're intended to treat. Antihistamines are notorious for sedation and fatigue, with other side effects including blurred double vision, changes in bowel habits, cognitive defects, dizziness, dry mouth/nose, ringing ears, stomach upset, and weakness. Not everyone experiences all of these side effects, and some people tolerate antihistamines better than others, so their use should be individualized.

Many of today's most effective antihistamines are coupled with a decongestant such as pseudoephedrine, thereby delivering a potent one-two punch against allergy symptoms. Some of the more popular new, less-sedating antihistamines include cetirizine (Zyrtec), fexofenadine (Allegra), and loratadine (Claritin) with common antihistamine/decongestant combinations being Claritin-D and Allegra-D, both with pseudoephedrine.

Older antihistamines like diphenhydramine (Benadryl) tend to be more sedating and are occasionally added to over-the-counter cold medications such as Excedrin PM or Extra Strength Tylenol PM to help people with colds and flu sleep. Diphenhydramine should never be used by people with narrow-angle glaucoma or an obstructed bladder.

The most dangerous side effect of antihistamines is the irregular and dangerous heart rhythms that were reported with astemizole (Hismanal) and terfenadine. The potentially fatal rhythm is called "torsades de pointes" and can occur if these agents are taken by people with liver disease, or used with certain antibiotics or antifungals. While most people can tolerate antihistamines, they are drugs with potentially dangerous side effects and drug-drug interactions, and should be used only under the care of a physician.

## Decongestants

Oral and nasal decongestants reduce blood flow to the nasal membranes, thereby relieving nasal congestion and stuffiness. One of the most popular decongestants is pseudoephedrine, which, as you may recall, was derived from the herb *Ephedra sinica*. Like antihistamines, oral decongestants are associated with several disturbing potential side effects, including constipation, dizziness, dry mouth/ nose, fatigue, irregular heart rhythms, palpitations, and sedation, and should be used only under the guidance of a doctor.

Topical decongestants containing oxymetazoline hydrochloride or phenylephrine hydrochloride (Afrin) tend to have fewer side effects, but they should not be used for more than three days as they have a paradoxical rebound phenomenon and can ultimately lead to increased nasal congestion. Overuse of topical decongestants can also injure the nasal lining, resulting in a painful condition called rhinitis medicamentosa. Other topical decongestant side effects include burning, sneezing, and stinging. Decongestants should not be used in people with diabetes, glaucoma, heart disease, or hyperthyroidism.

## Anticholinergics, Expectorants, and Bronchodilators

Anticholinergics work by reducing blood flow into the nasal tissue, thereby reducing nasal secretions. Because of their many side effects, which can include cognitive dysfunction, poor coordination, and vision changes, the Food and Drug Administration (FDA) determined in 1985 that anticholinergics should no longer be available over the counter to treat allergic symptoms. There are several nasal sprays, available by prescription only (Atrovent, for example) that are used to treat allergic and nonallergic rhinitis.

**Expectorant**
*Found in many over-the-counter cough preparations, this is a general term for any agent that is used to help loosen respiratory secretions.*

Expectorants help bring up secretions from the lungs and have little, if any, role in the treatment of allergies. Bronchodilators dilate the airways and are not indicated for the vast majority of people with allergies unless they have asthma or allergic asthma.

## Mast Cell Stabilizers

As we learned in Chapter 2, histamine is the primary bad-boy allergy chemical substance in a number of immune system cells like basophils and mast cells. Mast-cell stabilizers, such as cromolyn sodium (Nasalcrom), prevent mast cells from releasing histamine and are especially helpful in people with allergies. Even better, they are considered safe and are available over the counter, which means you don't need a doctor's prescription. Being a synthetic flavonoid, Nasalcrom acts as a bridge between a nutrient and a drug.

Since mast-cell stabilizers can take six weeks to work, they are intended for long-term control and are not useful for acute allergy symptoms. While their side-effect profiles tend to be low, occasional sneezing and stinging have been reported. Pharmacologically, the good news about mast-cell stabilizers is that no significant drug-drug interactions are currently reported.

## Steroids

Steroids (corticosteroids, glucocorticoids) are the most powerful allergy medications that dramatically reduce inflammation. This power, however, comes with a price, and all steroids, but especially the oral steroids, have the potential to demonstrate significant toxicity and side effects.

Nasal steroids, such as fluticasone propionate (Flonase), triamcinolone acetonide (Nasacort), mometasone furoate (Nasonex), and budesonide (Rhinocort) are, like antihistamines, the *therapy of last resort* for allergies. They are not normally prescribed for those with mild to moderate allergies, or symptoms that are brought on by specific and avoidable triggers. Since nasal steroids can take more than a week to work, they are not effective in aborting acute symptoms. While normally well tolerated when taken temporarily, in high dosages, these agents can still be absorbed into the blood and produce devastating side effects similar to those for oral steroids, such as glaucoma, growth retardation, and impaired wound healing. Other side effects include asthma, bloody nose, cough, headache, hoarseness, immune suppression, nasal burning/stinging/dryness, nasal septal perforation, nausea, sneezing, and sore throat. People who are at extra risk for serious side effects include children who can experience growth retardation, postmenopausal women not on hormone replacement, and individuals with inadequate dietary vitamin D and calcium. Nasal steroids should never be used in children under the age of six or during an acute nose infection.

Several steps can help prevent steroid-induced complications and these include using the lowest dose of nasal steroid possible and supplementing your diet with 1,000 mg of calcium and 400–800 IU of vitamin D daily to prevent osteoporosis. Unlike many antiallergy medications, the advantage of nasal steroids is that they lack significant drug-drug interactions when taken temporarily.

Oral steroids are only used to treat the most severe and potentially life-threatening allergic reactions, and even then are only used for several days. Oral steroids have no role in the chronic management of allergies and are only occasionally used for people with severe allergy-induced asthma.

## Immunotherapy

Immunotherapy (desensitization, hyposensitization,

or allergy shots) involves the repeated injection of increasing amounts of allergen extracts into the skin in the hope of desensitizing the individual to that particular allergen. While the mechanisms behind immunotherapy remain the subject of intense debate, we do know that the procedure can help people with allergic rhinitis, allergic asthma, or a history of insect-sting hypersensitivity. Immunotherapy can also be especially beneficial for people who have persistent exposure to a known allergic trigger, such as dust mites or pollen.

Immunotherapy is not, however, without its risks and people can experience allergic and, at times life-threatening, anaphylactic reactions to allergy shots. Another drawback is that immunotherapy often takes, at a bare minimum, four to five years to complete and the duration of benefits cannot be predicted after the therapy is finished. Further complicating matters is that some people may actually experience a worsening of symptoms once the therapy is finished, thereby necessitating the prospect of resuming the injections most people find painful. While immunotherapy may sound splendid on paper, the results are mixed at best. The most successful outcomes of immunotherapy are seen in children with allergies to dust and grass.

# CONCLUSION

I hope this book has helped you learn about allergies and how to prevent them. Perhaps the most important take-home message is that, for most people, allergies are preventable. Go through your home and make a list of the allergens you know have triggered an attack in the past and, if possible, rid these items from your home. Take control of your allergies—don't allow your allergies to take control of you! Much of the advice in this book can be used to make your home and life healthier. A proper diet, coupled with the judicious use of supplements, can help you add healthy years to your life and, equally important, be a component in living healthy.

What I mean by living healthy is embracing a program of a healthy diet, adequate sleep, regular exercise, and a balanced, positive outlook toward life that will enable you to enjoy many active and trouble-free decades. Allergies do not occur in a vacuum. Rather, for many, they are part of everyday life, and to beat them, it is important to learn, once again, how to live. If you learn to control your life and embrace a daily program of healthy living, you will not only overcome your allergies, but will also become the master of your own destiny. For most, allergies are a preventable medical condition. With the help of this book, you can potentially rid your life of allergies and enjoy the symptom-free life you so richly deserve.

# SELECTED
# REFERENCES

Bagnato, A, Brovedani, P, Comina, P, et al. Long-term treatment with thymomodulin reduces airway hyperresponsiveness to methacholine. *Annals of Allergy*, 1989; 62:425–428.

Bjorneboe, A, Soyland, E, Bjorneboe, GE, et al. Effect of dietary supplementation with eicosapentaenoic acid in the treatment of atopic dermatitis. *British Journal of Dermatology*, 1987; 117:463–469.

Bjorneboe, A, Soyland, E, Bjorneboe, GE, et al. Effect of n-3 fatty acid supplement to patients with atopic dermatitis. *Journal of Internal Medicine Supplement*, 1989; 225:233–236.

Bucca, C, Rolla, G, Oliva, A, et al. Effect of vitamin C on histamine bronchial responsiveness of patients with allergic rhinitis. *Annals of Allergy*, 1990; 65: 311–314.

Cavagni, G, Piscopo, E, Rigoli, E, et al. Food allergy in children: an attempt to improve the effects of the elimination diet with an immunomodulating agent (thymomodulin). A double blind clinical trial. *Immuno-pharmacology Immunotoxicology*, 1989; 11:131–142.

Ellwood, P, Asher, MI, Bjorksten, B, et al. Diet and asthma, allergic rhinoconjunctivitis and atopic eczema symptoms prevalence: an ecological analysis of the International Study of Asthma and Allergic Childhood (ISAAC) data. ISAAC Phase One Study Group. *European Respiratory Journal*, 2001; 17: 436–443.

Fogarty, A, Lewis, S, Weiss, S, et al. Dietary vitamin E concentrations, and atopy. *The Lancet*, 2000; 356: 1573–1574.

Genova, R, Guerra, A. Thymomodulin in management

of food allergy in children. *International Journal of Tissue Reactions*, 1986; 8:239–242.

Hu, FB, Bronner, L, Willett, WC, et al. Fish and omega-3 fatty acid intake and risk of coronary heart disease in women. *Journal of the American Medical Association (JAMA)*, 2002; 287:1815–1821.

Huang, SL, Lin, KC, Pan, WH. Dietary factors associated with physician-diagnosed asthma and allergic rhinitis in teenagers: analysis of the first Nutrition and Health Survey in Taiwan. *Clinical and Experimental Allergy*, 2001; 31:259–264.

Johnston, CS, Retrum, KR, Srilakshmi, JC. Antihistamine effects and complications of supplementing vitamin C. *Journal of the American Dietary Association*, 1992; 92:988–989.

Kasahara, T, Amemiya, M, Wu ,Y, et al. Involvement of central opioidergic and nonopioidergic neuroendocrine systems in the suppressive effect of acupuncture on delayed type hypersensitivity in mice. *International Journal of Immunopharmacology*, 1993; 15:501–508.

Korting, HC, Schafer-Korting, M, Klovekorn, W, et al. Comparative efficacy of hamamelis distillate and hydrocortisone cream in atopic eczema. *European Journal of Clinical Pharmacology*, 1995; 48:461–465.

Kouttab, NM, Prada, M, Cazzola, P. Thymomodulin: biological properties and clinical applications. *Med Oncology and Tumor Pharmacotherapy*, 1989; 6:5–9.

Lai, X. Observation on the curative effect of acupuncture on type I allergic disease. *Journal of Tradi - tional Chinese Medicine*, 1993; 13:243–248.

Lovell, CR, Burton, JL, Horrobin, DF. Treatment of atopic eczema with evening primrose oil. *The Lancet*, 1981; I, 278.

Marshall, PS, Colon, EA. Effects of allergy season on mood and cognitive function. *Annals of Allergy*, 1993; 71:251–25.

Mittman, P. Randomized double-blind study of freeze-dried Urtica dioica in the treatment of allergic rhinitis. *Planta Medica,*1990; 56:44–47.

Nelson, HS, Hirsh, SR, Ohman, JL, et al. Recommendations of the use of residential air cleaning devices in the treatment of allergic respiratory diseases. *Journal of Allergy and Clinical Immunology*, 1988; 82:661–669.

Ogle, KA, Bullock, JD. Children with allergic rhinitis and/or bronchial asthma treated with elimination diet. *Annals of Allergy*, 1977; 39:8–11.

Podoshin, L, Gertner, R, Fradis, M. Treatment of rhinitis with ascorbic acid solution. *Ear Nose Throat Journal*, 1991; 70:54–55.

Schalin-Karrila, M, Mattila, L, Jansen, CT, et al. Evening primrose oil in the treatment of atopic eczema: effect on clinical status, plasma phospholipid fatty acids and circulating blood prostaglandins. *British Journal of Dermatology*, 1987; 117:11–19.

Shivpuri, DN, Menon, MPS, Prakash, D. A crossover double-blind study on Tylophora indica in the treatment of asthma and allergic rhinitis. *Journal of Allergy*, 1969; 43:145–150.

Stewart, AC, Thomas, SE. Hypnotherapy as a treatment for atopic dermatitis in adults and children. *British Journal of Dermatology*, 1995; 132:778–783.

Storms, MD, Meltzer, EO, Nathan, RA, et al. Allergic rhinitis: the patient's perspective. *Journal of Allergy and Clinical Immunology*, 1997; 99:825–828.

Swoboda, M, Meurer, J. Treatment of atopic dermatitis with Hamamelis ointment. *British Journal of Phyto-therapy*, 1991/2; 2:128–32.

Tollesson, A, Frithz, A. Borage oil, an effective new treatment for infantile seborrheic dermatitis. *British Journal of Dermatology*, 1993; 25:95.

Villani, F, Comazzi, R, DeMaria, P, et al. Effect of dietary supplementation with polyunsaturated fatty acids on bronchial hyperreactivity in subjects with seasonal asthma. *Respiration*, 1998; 65:265–269.

Wright, S, Burton, JL. Oral evening primrose oil improves atopic eczema. *The Lancet*, 1982; ii:1120– 1122.

Zuskin, E, Lewis, AJ, Bouhuys, A. Inhibition of histamine-induced airway constriction by ascorbic acid. *Journal of Allergy and Clinical Immunology*, 1973; 51:218–226.

# OTHER BOOKS AND RESOURCES

Braly, J, Thompson, J. *Food Allergy Relief.* New York, NY: McGraw-Hill Professional, 2000.

Ivker, RS. *Sinus Survival: The Holistic Medical Treatment for Sinusitis, Allergies, and Colds.* New York, NY: Putnam Publishing Group, 2000.

Jones, MH. *The Allergy Self-Help Cookbook: Over 325 Natural Food Recipes Free of All Common Food Allergens: Wheat-Free, Milk-Free, Egg-Free, Corn-Free, Sugar-Free.* Emmaus, PA: Rodale Press, 2001.

May, JC. *My House is Killing Me!: The Home Guide for Families with Allergies.* Baltimore, MD: Johns Hopkins University Press, 2001.

Ogren, TL. *Allergy-Free Gardening: A Revolutionary Guide to Healthy Landscaping.* Berkeley, CA: Ten Speed Press, 2000.

Rapp, DJ. *Is This Your Child?: Discovering and Treating Unrecognized Allergies in Children and Adults.* New York, NY: HarperCollins, 1992.

### GreatLife Magazine
Consumer magazine with articles on vitamins, minerals, herbs, and foods.
*Available for free at many health and natural food stores.*

### Let's Live Magazine
Consumer magazine with emphasis on the health benefits of vitamins, minerals, and herbs.

Customer service:

1-800-676-4333

P.O. Box 74908

Los Angeles, CA 90004

*Subscriptions: 12 issues per year, $19.95 in the U.S.; $31.95 outside the U.S.*

### Physical Magazine

Magazine oriented to body builders and other serious athletes.

Customer service:

1-800-676-4333

P.O. Box 74908

Los Angeles, CA 90004

*Subscriptions: 12 issues per year, $19.95 in the U.S.; $31.95 outside the U.S.*

### The Nutrition Reporter™ newsletter

Monthly newsletter that summarizes recent medical research on vitamins, minerals, and herbs.

Customer service:

P.O. Box 30246

Tucson, AZ 85751-0246

e-mail: jack@thenutritionreporter.com

www.nutritionreporter.com

*Subscriptions: $26 per year (12 issues) in the U.S.; $32 U.S. or $48 CNC for Canada; $38 for other countries.*

## Allergy Support Groups

Having allergies can be hard and it may be helpful to talk to people who share your misery. Several allergy support groups available for adults and children with allergies are listed below.

***Parents of Allergic Children*** in Richmond, Virginia has a great website filled with useful information on many allergy-related subjects, such as attention deficit hyperactivity disorder (ADHD), ear infections, and food sensitivities. The website also contains a message board and chat room.

### Parents of Allergic Children
P.O. Box 1808
Midlothian, VA 23113
http://www.parentsofallergicchildren.org

### Parents of Food Allergic Kids
http://www.groups.yahoo.com/group/POFAK/

### The Allergy Discussion Group
An online resource for adults with allergies.
http://www.immune.com/allergy/index.html

### The Asthma Allergy Foundation of America
http://www.aafa.org

### Allergy Resources International
http://www.allergy.net/articles/index.cfm/html

## Suppliers of Allergy-Related Products

### The Allergy Buyers Club
161 North Street
Newtonville, MA 02460
Phone: 1-888-236-7231 • Fax: 1-617-332-0292
Website: http://www.AllergyBuyersClub.com

### Allergy Supply Company
11994 Star Court
Herndon, VA 20171
Phone: 1-800-323-6744 • Fax: 1-703-391-2014
Website: http://www.allergysupply.com

### Allergy One
P.O. Box 28302
Fresno, CA 93729-8302
Phone: 1-559-432-1900 • Fax: 1-559-432-1910
Website: http://www.allergyone.com
Email: allergyone@hotmail.com

# INDEX